Seeking Freedom and Joy
in the Winding Path of Life

Seeking Freedom and Joy in the Winding Path of Life

A Spiritual Journey of Learning and Self-Discovery

Antonietta Francini, M.D.

iUniverse, Inc.
New York Lincoln Shanghai

Seeking Freedom and Joy in the Winding Path of Life
A Spiritual Journey of Learning and Self-Discovery

iUniverse books may be ordered through booksellers or by contacting:

iUniverse
2021 Pine Lake Road, Suite 100
Lincoln, NE 68512
www.iuniverse.com
1-800-Authors (1-800-288-4677)

The views expressed in this work are solely those of the author and do not necessarily reflect the views of the publisher, and the publisher hereby disclaims any responsibility for them.

ISBN: 978-0-595-42531-0 (pbk)
ISBN: 978-0-595-86860-5 (ebk)

Printed in the United States of America

For my children
And in memory of my great Teachers

"All things are as they are,
As in no other way can they BE"

(Anonymous)

Contents

List of Pictures

Preface

I live now in rural Ontario, Canada. My house is surrounded by twenty acres of beautiful forest with wild life, deer, raccoons, and lots of birds. During all my life, I have been a medical doctor, a researcher, a scientist, and a mystic.

The desire of my lifetime was to see a bridge between science and mysticism. Finally, recently the new physics, chemistry and biology, are approaching the most essential concepts of mysticism. The science of quantum physics and the philosophy of universal consciousness are getting more and more linked in the questioning of the mysteries of the universe.

I want to share with you the lessons that I learned.

I realized that: "Intelligent-Cosmic-Consciousness, all Nature surrounding us, our physical body, and our intention/free will, are ONE and the same."

THAT is the Light that gives light to the stars!

All is entangled, related, connected to everything else.

All is glorious Life shining in a perfect cosmic dance in which we are the artists and the co-creators.

We are Divine manifestations. Nothing is separate; all is linked to everything else.

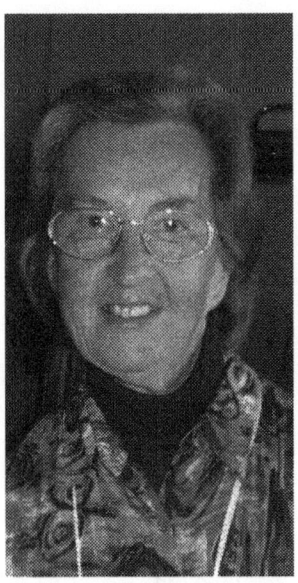

Introduction

I decide to publish this manuscript because the lessons that I learned are valuable for most people. It is our duty to share the sad and the good of every-days' life and to explain how we can overcome difficulties and take advantage of our experience to help others.

This book is about the challenges that crossed my path and how it was possible to overcome them emerging in peace and serenity in old age.

It is useful to understand that there are constant changes in everything. For example, an Italian popular saying states that: "There is no pain lasting hundred years." It means that whatever happens to you, it will not last long. We cannot be always happy, or always unhappy. Life has its own rhythm that alternates the good and the not so good. Just go with the flow, or go with the Tao, as the ancient Chinese wisdom advises.

The major aspects that shape the invisible background of my life story derive from the certainty that only *true spiritual evolution* grants us the fulfillment of our incarnation.

Life is about self-awareness and discipline. We must be able of setting clear goals and have a deep felt motivation. We should never undervalue the power of our thoughts and intentions! What we think we become! Remember that thoughts and subtle energies are the only "one-thing" faster then light!

I certainly had a well-defined goal when I studied to become a medical doctor. However, during my years of university I had a social and economic difficult time. I was alone in a distant country, short of money and often under the spell of 'post-traumatic-stress-disorder' (as this condition is defined in modern terms). Memories of the cruelties of World War II, of the bombings and the vision of wounded soldiers, would pop up in my mind on the occasion of every new stressful situation. This unpleasant disorder started during the war when I was a teenager and continued on and off for many years. Finally, it completely disappeared, with the blessings of my Guru Swami Muktananda Paramahamsa, when I went to India.

This is not the only characteristic in my life. There are others. One of them is related to open spaces and simple, primitive lifestyle. During several years, I experienced the profound healing power of mountains, deserts, and seashore. I learned more about natural life when I was a rural doctor caring for some indigenous tribes in South America. Getting deeply in touch with Nature, breathing pure fresh air and sweating under the tropical sun, are activities that nurture and heal body and mind. I felt myself alive, full of vitality and of joy for belonging to Mother Earth, to the sky full of stars, to the wind and to the storms!

My other trait is a keen interest for scientific research. I want to know, I want to be constantly updated on what goes on in physics, biology and mathematics. This interest has been very useful, as I am now able to link the recent theories of cosmic laws, of quantum physics and of mathematical formulas to the practical aspects of every day's life. I think that the modern research on 'free energy' and on Vibrational medicine is very interesting for everyone. I practice Holistic and Vibrational Medicine and often give instructional talks on these topics.

The other deep, very personal desire is my spontaneous tendency toward mysticism. I was born a mystic and since I was a child, the inner relationship with the Divine was natural to me. I still remember watching the blue sky from my open window and experiencing the presence of a cosmic goodness. This wonderful relationship with a superior being was suddenly interrupted when the rough reality of the cruel war hit my awareness. I could not understand why everything had changed so suddenly. The sky was the same blue sky, but now killing bombs were falling from it. Why? Where is my benevolent Being gone? Why did he disappear? No one around me could understand the deep reality of my anguish because nobody knew about my natural mystical tendency. I did not know it myself. I was so open to absorb Love, that when 'hatred' hit me, I got lost in doubts. These doubts also lasted many years and only by the Grace of the practice of the Science of Yoga, I was able to gradually dismiss them. The final big change occurred in India with the blessings of my Guru Swami Muktananda Paramahamsa.

We are constantly on a path of learning and discovery, of growing in wisdom and evolving in understanding, even if we must undergo the alternating struggles of "times of war and times of peace!"

This book is written in my 'fourth' language. Don't expect linguistic perfection! Just enjoy the flavour of my 'accent' and the sincerity of the story!

Antonietta Francini, M.D.
Practitioner of Holistic and Vibrational Medicine,
Ottawa, Canada, April 15, 2007

First Part:

War and Peace in My Early Life

Times of War:
My Struggles in Italy

I was born in Rome in a stormy day

I was born because my father wanted a boy, after having two girls in a previous marriage. He wanted a boy to continue the name and the business of the family, as he was a rich and powerful man. During the early 1920s in Italy, it was customary that a married woman used the husband's family name and played a submissive role in society. Women were not even allowed to have a personal bank-checking account! Therefore, my father, having only daughters, was condemned, not only to loose his family name in future generations, but also to pass on his remarkable fortune to a stranger, a will-be son in-law. That idea worried him greatly.

My mother was a teacher. She was twenty years younger and eager to please him. There was a great excitement about the future birth of a boy. The new-wed couple took residence in Rome, the capital, and my father, who was an architect, got into business investing in the construction market.

My mother organized the beautiful new house and started to hire attendants for the kitchen and the cleaning. The choice for a cook fell on a tall and strong, middle-aged woman who had very god references from a previous job. Her name was Adeline. She was illiterate, so, she could not read recipes, but she could certainly prepare delicious dishes. Besides, as she had previous experiences raising children, she would take care of the baby that was to be born a few months later.

The delivery took place in the house, attended by a skilled nurse.

On the due date the contractions started and a long difficult labour began. It was the end of November and a bad storm was blowing outside. Such harsh weather was exceptional for the usually mild climate of Rome and added anguish to the long, painful labour. The strong, blowing wind, bringing ice pellets and snow, continued unabated into the evening. Finally, around 4,30 pm, the last few dramatic moments of the baby's descent and expulsion, were expressed by a long desperate cry of intense suffering, victory and liberation!

The nurse announced loud: "Baby is healthy, it is a girl and is not breathing yet!" Another desperate cry followed the deception that it was not a boy, just another girl! What a shame!

Immediately after the delivery of the baby, a heavy haemorrhage got all the attention of the nurse and the new born, still not breathing, was dropped on a nearside bed. The baby was asphyxiating; became blue, and was going to die unattended.

Adeline was in the same room watching the delivery. She quickly understood that something had to be done fast, or it would be too late for the baby to survive. She had grown up in a farm and she knew what to do when a newborn calf or horse could not breath. She acted at once. Grabbing me by the feet, a blue, limp body with head and arms hanging down, she rushed to the terrace door and opened it wide, letting the storm blow into the house.

She jumped out on the terrace, grasped some snow in her hand, and started rubbing it on my back. That was an extreme reanimation treatment, but it worked! Life entered the still body with a loud cry and the first breath!

My life was offered to Mother Nature, to the storm, to the wind, and to the night, by the decisive action of a magic woman.

Adeline remained forever my real mother.

I learned about all this when I was about 6 years old. Adeline herself told me, and later my mother confirmed the story of my first breath.

I grew up a lonely child, as my parents did not want to risk another failure. Very early, I knew that I was not wanted, as I overheard a conversation; but, I could not understand what was wrong with me for not being a "boy."

Anyhow, I thought that something must be seriously wrong with me. I decided that I better kept silent and by myself. Only when I could run to the kitchen and embrace Adeline, my heart would expand with joy; but, that was only when my parents were not at home.

Later, when I went to school and was able to teach Adeline to read and write, our relationships became very close. We learned together, doing the same homework and reading the same children's books.

The story of Adeline

As a child, I was curious, I wanted to know; I was not afraid of facing the mysteries of the world of adults. When I was with Adeline in the kitchen, listening to the stories of her life, I knew that it was real life and that the stories written in the books were invented, just like the tales about witches and ogres.

Adeline grew up in the countryside as the older daughter in a very poor family. As a child, she had to go to the river and wash the clothes of the family. I could imagine her as myself carrying heavy loads and going to the cold river early in the morning, kneeling on the riverbank and washing clothes on a stone. Adeline had a bad scare on her left thumb because, when she was very young, their old house collapsed during one winter night. It caught fire and she was rescued from the ruins when her hand was already on fire.

She knew a lot about raising animals and about plants. She would tell me stories about forests, trees and storms, about her fears and about her good times when she was a child at her village. She never went to school, but together with me she learned to read and write. We had a great time together.

From Adeline's stories, I learned to adapt to the environment, as she used to tell me:

"There is no point on fighting when you have to obey. Understand that we have to accept the reality and the evidence of facts. I am poor and I have worked at the service of others all my life," she would say, "but nobody has put me down. I am independent and I know who I am."

I understood what it meant to be self sufficient even if apparently dependent on others. At that time, I certainly was not aware of the important lessons that I received from her, but later on, I understood better her wisdom.

It was only later, during the difficult years of the war, that I could fully understand the greatness of Adeline's soul. With her example, I learned courage and optimism during the worst moments. A strong, permanent, unconditional love emanated steadily from all her being. She was always open, trusting, giving, and receiving. I am alive because of her daring gesture, because of her impulse and inspiration, because she obeyed the will of Mother Nature and saved a life!

She could have lost her job, or she could have been accused of killing me for exposure to the cold. It could have been just a second too late! She risked a jail sentence to save my life! Her generosity, her spontaneous love for a baby made her act as a real Mother, no matter what the risk for herself could have been.

Destiny wanted that baby to live. The thunderstorm raged for hours over the city, the ice collected over the terrace, Adeline was present and followed the call of her generous heart in the most selfless gesture of risking her life for mine!

My early years

I started primary school at age six in an institute run by German Nuns. There, in the chapel, I found for the first time a beautiful statue of Jesus the Sheppard. It was a white marble statue showing a young boy with a sheep across his shoulders. It impressed me profoundly in his attitude of gentle benevolence and service. From then on he was my best friend, in my dreams and in my long solitary conversations before falling asleep.

When I was about 7 years old, an Austrian young lady came to live in our house and was my teacher of German. Her name was Anne. She lived in the house for a couple of years helping Adeline with house chores, walking me to school and taking me for walks during the weekends. She was tall, thin, very blond, and very religious. She did her best to teach me to always keep the company of Jesus in my mind. She was a great companion and I loved her very much. Naturally, one day my mother got jealous and suddenly she kicked her out. The loss of this friend was devastating for me.

I remember a story that Anne used to illustrate her teachings.

There was once a boy whose mother was very sick, but he was sure that Jesus could tell him what to do for restoring her health. So, he went to his grandfather and asked:
"What shell I do to talk with Jesus?"
The grandfather said:
"You must sit very quiet and still, and call Him. Then, you wait, without thinking on anything, just be silent, waiting for the answer. He will tell you what to do."
The boy was happy with the old mans' advice. He sat near the fireplace and from the depth of his heart, he called Jesus to help his mother and tell him what to do. After a little while he put a new log into the fire, then started to play with a stick, always waiting for an answer. But, no answer came. He was disappointed, but the next evening he started again calling for help. Again, he fixed the fire and played with a stick. Receiving no answer, he returned to his grandfather very sad. The old man asked:
"Were you doing something while you were waiting?"
"Yes, said the boy, I was fixing the fire and I had a stick to play with."
"No,—said the old man,—you are supposed to be absolutely still, do nothing and just wait for the answer to your call. Don't do anything and don't think on anything."
Finally the boy understood that in order to receive an answer from Jesus you must be concentrated with great attention on expecting an answer and don't be distracted by other activities. By following this advice he finally received the answer he expected and his mother was cured.

Anne told me this story several times insisting that I understood what it meant to be absolutely still and wait for an answer from Jesus. I loved her very much because I felt that she loved me and that this teaching was important for her. I did not know how important this advice would be later in my life.

This is how I received my first instructions on how to meditate when I was just about eight years old. Later I learned that the capacity of maintaining an absolute stillness and a vivid hope of communication with the Divine is the foundation of meditation. In later years, this practice would save my life. During the time of war, Anne's memory and the practice she taught me helped me go through many fears and difficult moments.

From Adeline and from Anne, I derived all the concepts about how to live a proper life. Both always told me:

To respect and obey my parents and my teachers,
To be sincere at all cost and in any circumstance,
To perform my duties the best I could,
To remain by myself and don't mix too much with people, and mostly,
To talk with God and trust His guidance.

These five rules were deeply established in me during my early years by the loving presence of these two women. On this solid foundation, I built my life in trust. Respect and obedience, sincerity, responsibility, dignity, and God guidance supported me during severe hardships and helped me face all problems.

Shortly after Anna left our house and went back to her home in Austria, I had the opportunity to find another friend who became very important in my life. It was during the summer of 1934. One day, when I was playing in the garden of my house, a young boy about ten years old came to the fence and begged for some bread.

"Yes, I will get it for you!" I said.

I went up to my apartment and got some fresh bread in the kitchen. The boy was very hungry and ate it with great enthusiasm. Then, we started to talk and he told me that he had three siblings but they were very poor because the father died and the little money that the mother was making was not sufficient for all. So, I promised that I would save some food for him and he started to come every day to meet me at the fence.

We became good friends and from our conversations, I learned a lot about the real life of poor people. I felt that it was similar to the kind of life Adeline had to endure when she was very young. She was a survivor of tragedies, poverty, and family hardships in her own hometown.

The contrast with my own life as a rich girl was a hard lesson for me. I felt a stronger relationship with poor people than with my own parents. My mother and father were both somehow alien to my feelings. I loved Adeline, Anna, and now this little boy, begging at the fence. They were all poor people. With them, I felt love, sincerity, connection, freedom of feelings and of speech. On the contrary, every intent of relationship with my own parents was with effort and artificial. I just did not like it and very early, I rejected that type of social, conventional world that they considered appropriate.

The summer months passed quickly and I went back to school. Therefore, I was not able to see my little friend again. One day I was in the kitchen doing my homework with Adeline, when the doorbell rang. I answered the call, opened the door and there was my little friend sad and hungry. I put a finger on my lips to signal him not to speak, but to wait there. I run back to the kitchen to get some bread and a couple of oranges, but, on my way to the door, both my parents emerged from another room into the corridor. I quickly hurried to give the boy his food signalling him to run away and closed the front door.

But, my parents asked what was I doing and who was at the door. "Nobody, it was a mistake, someone looking for another family!" I said.

"Why did you give them oranges?"

"Because the boy was hungry!"

"So, you are feeding beggars?!! Never do that again! Beggars are not allowed to come to this house! If they show up again, the police will be notified!"

"But the boy is hungry!"

"That's none of your business! Beggars are people who don't want to work, and should be punished for not working, they are lazy and irresponsible! You don't have anything to do with beggars! Do you understand?"

"And now, go to your room and never open the front door again!

Adele, do you understand? The girl is never to open the front door again.

Beggars will not be given anything and if they insist, call the police!"

I remember this episode as a cornerstone in my life! My parent's words hit me in the stomach like a thunderstorm with flashes of lightning. All my love for my only little friend was smashed into pieces and forbidden forever! At that moment, I understood what "social" conditioning is all about. Immediately I knew that I would never belong to that kind of society. I went to my room, knelt beside a chair, and took the most serious and profound vow of all my life. I still remember almost exactly the words I used to formulate it:

"Jesus, my Lord, I promise that I will dedicate all my life, my power and my attention only to help the poor. Whatever I will do, it will only be useful to help the poor. I never want to be rich and selfish. This commitment is for all my life. Help me realize this promise! Amen."

Then I meditated asking Jesus to help me cope with the negative feelings that I felt for my parents. I also made a detailed plan to keep my intention secret. I could not involve Adeline in my decision because she could be sent away at any moment, if my parent got jealous of her or suspected my dislike for them. So, I had to present and indifferent face, keep my secret for myself, and protect Adeline who was the only living creature that I loved and who loved me.

Looking back, I recognize that it was a terribly stressful moment for me and it brought serious consequences. Shortly after I became critically ill with an infection of the tonsils that spread to my entire body and damaged the kidneys. I had high fever, my face and hands were swollen, and I had albumin in the urine. No antibiotics were available at that time. The only treatment was bed rest and no-salt diet. I remained in bed-rest for more than six months. I remember lying flat on my back and watching for hours the small white clouds crossing the sky outside of my window.

Children's books and dolls did not help me in my solitude and boredom. So, one day that my parents were not at home and Adeline was busy in the kitchen, I jumped out of bed and went to search for some interesting books in the large bookcases in my parent's studio-room. There were lots of books, two walls of them, hundreds of volumes, all thick, hardcover and imposing. I was looking for something that I could handle and hide under the mattress, something easy to read, and interesting. My hands worked their way behind large volumes and I felt some small and soft pages hidden in the back of the imposing books. That was what I was looking for! Immediately I knew that those pages were what I was searching. Carefully, I removed the small hand-typed booklets from their hiding place and with a sense of victory, I carried them close to my chest until I jumped back in bed.

What a finding! They were booklets on Yoga, by Yogi Ramacharaka and carried the date of the printing: 1904. The first was a series of lessons on breathing exercises, the other was titled "14 Lessons on the Philosophy of Yoga," and the third was titled "Mystic Christianity." I new nothing about Yoga, but immediately I felt a great joy, like if I had found a great, long forgotten friend.

Now, I had something to read, something to do, practicing the breathing exercises and it was something that would certainly help my recovery.

After a few months of reading and practicing Yoga in my solitary confinement, the doctor found that my kidneys were recovering. No more albumins, no more infection, and no more oedemas. The doctor permitted me to get out of bed and sit on a chair. My diet of milk and boiled potatoes without salt improved with the addition of one apple a day.

That apple made all the difference in the world. As Yogi Ramacharaka suggested in his book, I concentrated on thinking that by eating the apple I was absorbing the energies of the Sun and of Mother Earth. The apple was the product of a healthy apple tree, tall and proud in the Sun and in the wind. A visiting bee had pollinated the flowers and the apple had grown slowly under the warm rays of our benevolent Star! All the Cosmic energies of Life were concentrated in the modest apple that I was slowly chewing.

Those teaching were very influential to shape my life. It was the winter of 1934, just past my ninth birthday. A big decision about my future started to grow inside me inspired by the wise teachings of the booklets. I felt that I wanted to become a medical doctor to help suffering people and that I would follow the methods illustrated in those pages, both, to reinforce my own health, and to help others. I did not imagine how truth that insight would become about twenty years later. I am forever grateful to my great teacher Yogi Ramacharaka and to his instructions that helped my fast recovery, not only in that first encounter, but also thirty years later when the cancer hit.

Shortly after, my health recovered completely. I returned to school and my life went back to normal.

Arriving from school one day, I had a surprise.

Adeline opened the door of our apartment to let me in and told me:

"Your mother wants to talk to you, she is in the studio."

"Why? What happened?"

"Nothing serious, but she is sad!"

I gave my school bag to Adeline and went to the studio.

My mother was sitting at the desk and on top of it were my precious booklets of Yoga by Ramacharaka. Immediately I understood that the new cleaning lady had found them under my mattress.

"How did you get these books?" asked my mother very serious.

"I found them in the bookshelf."

"And why are you keeping them hidden in your bed?"

"Because I like them very much and I have been studying them and practicing the breathing exercises."

"But, you are too young to understand these teachings!"

"No, Mammy, they are very clear to me!"

She paused, took a deep breath and looked at me very serious:

"These are the last gift that I received from my fiancée before he went to war and died on the battlefield during World War I. They are a very dear and sad memory for me. He gave me these books to keep in the hope of coming back home, but he never did! He was a great friend of my father and was a Medical Doctor and a Mason, as my father was. They studied these books together and he wanted me to study them too, but I never did. We were going to get married at the end of the war. But, all my dearest ones died during those terrible years, my father, my two brothers, who were killed in the war and finally Umberto, my fiancée. He died of the wounds received in battle."

"So, his name is Umberto! I have been thinking so much on who could be the owner of these wonderful books! Now I know, his name: Umberto!"

"How old was he when he died, Mammy?"

"He was about twenty-six, he had just graduated and was going to start his practice with my father. That was terrible! Both died!"

My mother started to cry silently, overcome by emotion.

I felt suddenly that a new relationship had opened up between my mother and me; a new friendship, a new vision of who she really was; a new connection linked somehow to these books!

Only much, much later did I understand how everything had evolved. The memory of Umberto and his love for my mother; the image of Umberto being a medical doctor and studying yoga, kept returning to my mind. I realized that I was very interested in these books myself and that I had decided to become a medical doctor after studying the yoga teachings. I felt a great connection between Umberto, my mother, and my self.

These concepts evolved later in a much deeper understanding of the whole situation.

My father died in 1936. He decided to sell all his business and investments in construction before passing away. He believed that it was the best for us, for my mother and for me, to have money in the bank and not to have to care for rented buildings and real estate investments. He only kept the house where we were living.

He could not imagine that a few years later a terrible war would reduce us to extreme poverty. The value of the money fell to almost nothing and several banks closed for bankruptcy. How false are expectations about transitory goods!

The house where we were living was a seven-floor building with twelve apartments for rent. It could have given us some income, but the rents were frozen by law at the beginning of the war in 1940. All we could get was the value corresponding to one egg a month, at the prices of the black market. My father had good intentions, but the political reality, just four years after his death, made us very poor.

After my father died, my mother decided to send me to public school. The environment was very strange and new to me. Looking back at that first year in public school, I don't know how I could stand it. I had no idea how to socialize and how to deal with other girls and boys. They were like aliens from another planet and so I must have been for them. I had no idea what they were talking about. The topics and the expressions they used were very new to me. In order to save myself from ridicule I opted for talking as little as possible. This went on for a full academic year, but when the next term approached, I squarely refused to continue to study. I told my mother that I would not go to school any more. That was final. She got very angry but I was glad that she was mad at me, so she would leave me alone.

A few days later, Adeline asked me to help her with some shopping and we went together to the market place. Adeline did not really need any help, she was just furious with me and with my behaviour. She wanted to talk to me alone. The first thing she said was that I was selfish and lacked discrimination.

"Shame on you!" she said, "because some stupid girls may laugh at you, you decide to take such irresponsible decision!"

"Shame on you!" "Your duty is to study, to graduate, to go on to university and to be useful to others and to society! Now, just because of a fantasy you are going to fail to your duty! Shame on you!" "You will never forgive your self later in life, if you insist in this nonsense!"

Her words hit me right in the middle. She was right. How could I help others if I did not study? What about my secret promise? I lowered my head and started to cry right there, in the middle of the market place. I could not stand her reproaches!

Not only did I go back to school, but I also tried hard to be more social and to understand the mentality of my schoolmates. I even once went to a party in the house of one of the girls. That was the first and only time that I went to a party during my teen years. Then, Italy was forced to enter the war in 1940 because of the political alliance with Berlin.

Shortly after our life became hell.

When this happened, I returned to my dear solitude and to my very precious books. I continued high school practically by myself. During the war, the schools typically remained closed because of the bombings. I passed my final exams when I was seventeen, one year ahead of everyone else.

Immediately after, I registered in the school of Medicine at the University of Rome. We had no classes and the university was closed, but we had exams twice a year and I completed my third year after the end of the war.

When the war ended in 1945, we were penniless. Looking back, I remember how proud and successful my father was in business and how he so wanted a boy to carry on the estate. Twenty years later, his fortune was gone. His anxiety over a successor to the business meant nothing; there was no business, no money, and his family name would not last another generation. What a life lesson! Money and possessions come and go with the wind. Materialism is impermanent, only our inner development and stamina enable us to climb to the next stage of existence

World War II (1939-45)

> *The paranoia of two dictators and the sheepish Obedience of several million people caused Fifty two million deaths and the destruction of the entire European Continent.*

∧∧∧∧∧∧∧∧∧∧∧∧∧∧∧∧

Brief introduction-World War II in Europe-

At the beginning of the nineteen-century, a sequence of social disasters and discords in Europe brought about the First World War (1915-18).

The end of this war was followed by twenty years of dictatorships in different European Countries. There were four cruel dictators: one in Spain, one in Italy, one in Germany and one in Russia. Each of these dictators continued to brainwash their compatriots with ideas of hatred, revenge, and fear.

I remember that the discourses of Mussolini were daily voiced from loud speakers on top of government buildings: "We are the target of criminals that want to destroy us, … they hate us and we must hate them,…. who is not with us is against us,…. we must fight and take revenge, … we will destroy them, or they will destroy us, … be aware of the danger, … don't trust anybody, … the enemy is everywhere,…." and so on. Similar instigations continued during about twenty year all over Europe! The four dictators, in different languages were projecting their hatred on every citizen. Fear and aggression, the lowest human emotions, were strongly stimulated.

The large, dark, menacing cloud of thoughts of fear and hatred build up slowly but densely over Europe. The final terrible storm had to be apocalyptic because of the intensity of the power of dissolution. Thoughts have great power when repeated and condensed with the fear of million people. Therefore, the terrible consequences were overwhelming and began in 1939, when the Nazis invaded Poland.

For us, in Italy, the disaster started with a great political mistake: the alliance of Mussolini with Hitler. The Germans had been the enemies of the Italians for centuries.

Historically, the barbarians from the north invaded Italy and destroyed the Roman Empire in the fourth century. Invaders from the North always brought great destruction to our country. The Germans occupied the North of Italy during the nineteenth century and the population hated them.

When the Fascist government announced the alliance with the Nazis, the entire population was shocked. Germans were the enemies of Italy since ever. There were too many memories of abuses, of military occupation, of people tortured and killed. This could not be forgotten, nor forgiven by the Italian population.

My mother was furious. She was born in Verona, she and her family had suffered under the German military occupation before World War I. She had lost two brothers and her fiancée that were killed during the battle of Vittorio Veneto. In that battle, finally, the Italian army rejected the Germans across the Alpine Range. It was impossible for my mother to forgive Mussolini for such an unbelievable treason. She felt that the alliance with Germany was a treachery to the memory and to the sacrifice of her dear ones. This feeling was shared by most Italians of her generation.

The Fascist government was well aware of the public opposition against the alliance with the Nazis. A strong movement of rebellion against the Nazi's cruelty began when the news of the massacres of the Polish Jewish spread among us. We did not want to have bloody hands from the slaughter of children and civilians. The mass murder of Jews by gassing started in June 1942 in Auschwitz and in July of the same year, at the extermination camp of Treblinka.

Until that moment, the political propaganda had told us that a war was needed because of economical reasons. It was supposed to be related to the economic sanctions that the international markets had dictated against Italy. We were told that it had to do with international trade.

Since the beginning of the war in 1939, until 1942, it was more a question of Hitler invading Poland and Russia for reasons that in Italy no one could understand. We all predicted that he would fail, as Napoleon had failed. Our studies of history suggested that the terrible northern winter would take care of the invading armies, as it had in the past. We somehow expected that the defeat of the Nazis in Eastern Europe would be the end of the war. Our predictions were in part correct, the Nazis were defeated, but the war took a new turn in Africa.

Africa is very close to Italy toward the South.

The popular and political opposition grew stronger and firm, even if heavily repressed by the secret police. In January 1943, a complot was organized from the inside to overthrow the Fascist government. The conspirators were Ciano (who was the Foreign Minister), the Field Marshal Cavallero (who was the armed forces Chief of Staff), the Field Marshal Badoglio, and others. Inevitably, internal spies notified Mussolini, and he quickly replaced the armed forces Chief of Staff and fired Ciano. That was the beginning of the end for Fascism and for Italy. At that moment, Mussolini lost the support, not only of the general population, but of a large portion of the army as well.

Political tension started building up among the military between Germans and Italians. Boycott of military actions, self-sinking of ships, sabotages and destruction of military supplies, became common.

In Italy, all the syndicates and the factory workers were rebelling against Mussolini and against the wrong alliance with the Nazis. In March 1943, the aeronautics plant in Turin went on strike. The special fascist troops sent by Mussolini to stop the strike refused to force the workers to go back to work. The popular rejection for the Fascist regimen was so strong that their special troops opted for prison and torture, but did not act against the workers. Other strikes erupted, weakening the war making capacity of Fascism. Next, a series of boycotts destroyed several ships carrying troops and equipment to Tunisia for the continuation of the war in Africa.

I remember that after this internal resistance, it was clear that the government was crumbling. Documents found after the war show that Mussolini tried to convince Hitler to give up the war in Russia and to concentrate on the occupation of Africa, predicting that the loss of Africa would mean the invasion of Italy.

As predicted, in June 1943 the Allies paratroopers parachuted in Sicily and the invasion followed with landing crafts. We were not happy, but nor very afraid, thinking that the end had been reached.

It was clear that Italians did not want to be allied with the Nazis. We were just instruments of Hitler's lust for power. At that moment, it was also too late! Italy was completely under the dominion of Nazi's forces.

After establishing firmly their landing in Sicily in July 1943, the Allies started a heavy bombing of all the Nazis' positions. The first bombing of Rome occurred on July 19, 1943. It was a disaster with more than seven thousand deaths. We had never experienced such a heavy bombing before. That was the terrible beginning!

When this happened, finally, our short-sighted King, Vittorio Emanuele, understood something of what was going on and, in a rare moment of bright thinking, called Mussolini to a meeting at the royal palace in Rome and arrested him on July 25, 1943.

Mussolini was sent to jail in a military fortress. Shortly after, the Nazis rescued him and he survived two years more in the North of Italy.

Immediately after Mussolini's arrest, a terrible political confusion started.

The new government changed its political position three times in 1943:
in the month of July, Italy was declared allied with the Nazis;
in the month of September, Italy was declared neutral;
in the month of October, Italy declared war to his Nazis occupants.

The change in the political scene, from being allies of the Nazis to becoming politically neutral and occupied territory of the Nazis, and finally enemies of our occupants, left us civilians in terrible condition.

When that happened, we understood that we were in a real terrible danger. We faced an internal revolution together with a bloody war and an immediate Nazi military occupation. Absolutely no one would care for us, the innocent civilians. Can you imagine surviving without any public services? No electricity, no water, and no food, nothing to live on?

The Nazi officially occupied Rome as conquered territory. The freedom fighters started to act against the military occupation. The Nazis responded with terrible cruelty with tortures and killing of innocents grabbed from the streets or invading buildings and taking prisoners all the occupants, old people, children, and women. We expected to be taken to torture every day, watching from the window day and night. Others died for us.

It is difficult to find in history a modern government who did so much harm to its own population as the Italian rulers during World War II.

The new political rulers were the symbols of unbelievable incapacity and fear. Twenty years (from 1921 to 1943) of dictatorship had frozen their brains completely. People were not used to think, but only to obey orders. A whole generation of military chiefs was unable to think properly when they had to take important decisions. This shows that the destructive influence of dictatorship extends for generations.

Later I learned that this last unfortunate declaration of war against the Nazis, when Italy was already occupied, starving, and impotent, responded to the hope of being able of sitting at the peace table participating in the negotiations. It was a convenient political choice, but for us it was a tough time.

The war in Central and Northern Italy continued until May 2, 1945.

On April 28, 1945 Mussolini was captured and hanged by Italian partisans.

On April 30, 1945 Hitler committed suicide in Berlin

On May 7, 1945, all Nazi forces surrendered unconditionally to the Allies.

∧∧∧∧∧∧∧∧∧∧∧∧∧∧∧∧∧∧∧∧∧∧∧∧∧∧∧∧

My traumatic experiences of the war

The two long, dark years 1943-44 were extremely tough for us. Some times, during those terrible war years, I lost the notion of what it was like to have a normal life. I came to think that bombing, lack of food, of water, of electricity, of toilet paper and of all kind of commodities, was the usual way of life.

Death and misery were all around us. Refugees were flowing in from the countryside hoping to find some shelter in the city. Old people and young children were the only people left in the city, able men and women were all directly involved in the conflict.

Wounded German soldiers escaping from the horrors of the battlefield a few kilometres south of Rome were wandering in the streets before collapsing unattended in any corner. They were young teenagers almost my age, the last resources send south by the German Nazis to fight and die in Montecassino.

Most of the politicians responsible for getting us into the war were dead or had run away. The Nazis had invaded Italy and considered us as traitors. They had tortured and killed as many Italians as they could. I remember hearing during the night the screams of women and old men dragged to be tortured for the fun of some sadistic Nazis officer. We were completely defenceless. We were occupied enemy territory.

The final battle in the south of Italy lasted almost a year a hundred kilometres south of my house. We could hear the bombs, the shooting of the cannons, the clarity of the fires and the battle going on day and night. Thousand of young lives were lost in that carnage. Today a vast field of crosses is a reminder of the criminality, cruelty, and paranoia of dictators and of the sheepish obedience of several million people.

During the years 1943 and 1944 day and night the Allies were bombing the cities in the north of Italy, the railways and the surroundings of Rome. At dusk and during the night the skies were shaking with the deep sound of heavy bombers flying over my house in waves. Sometimes they would bomb a vast area close to the railway, a few blocks south of my house, and the walls and windows would shake with the explosions.

I clearly remember the typical terrifying sound of falling bombs. It is like a whistle that starts soft and high pitched and becomes louder, and low pitched when the bomb is about to hit. You can hear it, but you never know if it is close, or far enough from you. When you hear it, that is death coming down, but you never know if it will miss you or blow you up.

We did not go to the basement, nor sought protection. The best is to be killed on the spot. We stayed on the seventh floor of my house, in my mothers' room, waiting to die any day or night during that time. Other people used to go to the basement every time the alarm sounded, but that happened ten or more times during the twenty four hours and after a while you cannot cope with the stress of rushing up and down the stairs. Besides, the possibility of being trapped in a basement under a collapsed building and suffer a death by starvation is worst then being blown up immediately.

There was a large building, one of the few still standing a couple of blocks form my house where lots of refugees from the countryside and from the farmlands were crowded. One evening at eight the convoy of the Allied bombers came over us and hit that building heavily, no one knows why. The building crushed completely, the upper floor collapsing on top of the lower floors. The fortunate ones who were in the higher floors died a quick death, but those who were trapped in the lower floors had a terrible death from suffocation and starvation.

For about a week after the bombing we could hear the cries for help, the despair of the survivors trapped in the ruins, the slow agony of those who were entombed alive without hope. There was no equipment, no helpers, and no possibility of rescuing anybody. We had to stand the long hours of hopeless screaming and lamenting.

After a few weeks, when all sounds had stopped, the Pope came and gave his blessings to the ruins declaring it to be a holy burial ground.

I was there. Not a word was said about the insanity of the fact!

Unbelievable!

During the same time, our struggle for food and mostly for water was a daily obsession. We had to find the strength and the fortitude to go out of the house in search of some water; or we had to stand on line for unending hours during night and day to get some flour, hoping to make some bread and find somewhere a place to cook it! The three of us, Adeline, my mother, and myself would take turns for these tasks. Unfortunately, my mothers' cooperation was very little. She was depressed and stayed in bed most of the time after having an almost deadly experience; she hardly escaped with life after being shot by an Allied pilot at noontime on a city street.

This is how it happened.

One day, my mother was walking from our house to the cemetery; she used to go there to find some comfort from sitting beside my fathers' grave. Suddenly, she heard someone screaming behind her: "They are coming, jump into the ditch, now, fast!" and she was pushed violently at the side of the road by an old man. The man jumped beside her and the airplane came down low over them shooting automatic gunshots. The man was hit and died instantly bleeding profusely, just next to my mother in the ditch. She returned home bleeding herself, lightly wounded and terrified. No point in seeking help, as none could be found anyhow.

The emotional consequences were devastating for my mother and she only recovered at the end of he war.

Adeline would usually stand on line for food during the nights. My typical duty was mostly to find water every day. There were so called public fountains; they consisted of large metal tanks that were filled with some fluid called water, no question if clean or murky, located here or there in some square or street. If the water arrived during the night, one or two were open by the military police during the day. A long line-up started at dawn. Sometimes we were permitted to fill up two containers, but most of the time only one and some times the water was finished by the time you reached the end of the line. Then, there was the long walk home carrying the precious water. I built a little device using my skates, a wooden table, and a rope and I was able to carry two full buckets from very far away without too much effort.

One day on my trip home, I faced a very young, wounded, German soldier. I can still see his face. A child; he was a teenager like me. All the right side of his face and his uniform were stained with dried blood. He was standing in front of me staring at the water. He was my enemy. He was the invader and the torturer, but how could I refuse him water? He was dying. I had no small container, so he drank from my hands; he was feverish and very thirsty. Then he slowly walked away, hopeless and desperate. A cruel, solitary death awaited him, imposed by the Nazi dictatorship!

In that moment, I hated God! How could he permit so much suffering? His supposed love for humanity was only a tragic deception. Why did the Nuns tell me that god is love? Why did everybody lie to me? Why did Anne, my best friend, tell me fantastic stories of love and care? Why should children like that soldier be sent to kill and to be killed? Why was humanity so blind to the injustice? Why could a loving God permit such carnage of young lives?

This episode, the pain, the horror of the wounds and of the suffering stayed with me forever.

It was dangerous to walk on the streets during that time. The danger was both on the ground and from the air. The small airplanes, the fighters escorting the large Allied bombers flying north, had nothing to do because no German aircraft was challenging the huge bombers. So the pilots would take advantage of the fact that Rome had no organized aerial defence and would come down and have fun firing their machine gun on some passer-by, as they did with my mother. We were flesh for fun for everybody.

The other danger of being on the streets was due to the Nazis' constant effort for kidnapping whoever could walk. They needed slaves to work in their factories in the north. They would grab you and pack you with hundred others in a wagon trying to send you north, beyond the Alpine range. That was hopeless because the Allies would daily bomb all the trains, or you would starve inside the locked wagon during the trip. Nevertheless, Nazis always obeyed orders, so they kept kidnapping people in the south to send them north, even if no one could arrive alive during the last years of war.

They almost got me once.

As I was rounding a corner, I suddenly saw a big military truck unloading armed soldiers who were racing into the lateral streets to close in by surprise whoever was in that block of streets. I was able to escape from the opposite side! I could run really fast!

Nevertheless, no matter what the dangers, we had to be on the street every day in search for food and water! Like wild animals in the deep jungle!

Suddenly, something changed in the spring of 1944. The shootings of the battle between the advancing Allies and the resisting Nazi troops came closer. There were more injured wandering German soldiers everywhere. Groups of them. Obviously, the hospital services at the battlefront were unable to cope with the bombing and the wounded. Many soldier had serious injuries; some were missing arms or legs, soaked in blood, they were helping each other or abandoning those dying. We did not dare to go out at all. It was apocalyptic! A stream of dying souls erupting from hell! I could watch them from my window with a shiver hoping that they would not throw down my door in search of water or food, which we did not have anyhow.

After a few days, Adeline dared to go out. We needed water and we noticed some women rushing in the streets holding buckets. Adeline told me to stay at home and grabbed the pail. When she came home, she carried the precious water and told us the news.

The battle was over and the Allies were coming closer. The Nazis were desperate because their roads for the retreat toward the north were cut by the gunfire of the airplanes and the by the bombings. There was the possibility that they decided to hold on to Rome as their last defence, by fortifying the city and fighting in every building until the winter. We were terrified. That meant for us a horrible death.

Then, there was a pause. For a few days, some calm returned. We could get some flour and we ventured out of the city into the nearby countryside in search of dandelions and other herbs that were growing in the fields. Spring was generous and we collected a good amount of herbs and roots. Adeline had grown up in a farm and was an expert in detecting herbs that were good to make soup and safe to be consumed. We got some coal to put in the stove, some matches, and some paper to start the fire. Each one of these simple items was difficult to get, expensive and rare.

My mother had sold all of her rings, some jewellery, carpets, furniture; all that could be sold was given away to survive. But, we had survived! And that day, in the spring of 1944, we had a great soup with flour, herbs, and even some salt!

A few days later, I got a desperate message from a close friend of mine that had been kidnapped by the Nazis and whom we considered to be dead. He was a student of medicine like me. I had met him during one of the few exams that the university had scheduled during the last two years. He had been recruited to work in the military hospital in Rome and was one of the few young males walking in the streets. The Nazis got him and sent him in one of those horrible convoys going north.

His sister had given me the news of his capture and came again to my house with a cry for help. She told me that my friend had escaped from the convoy, that he had been walking along the bank of the river Tiber toward Rome, and that he was now hiding in some riverbank close to the city. He was in constant danger of being discovered and was starving. A young girl, searching for dandelions and flowers to eat, had found him and informed her mother about him and his home address. The woman had walked several kilometres to notify the family of my friend about his escape and his hiding.

The older and the younger sisters of my friend came to see me for help. The young man was too weak to walk away from his hiding place and it was not safe for him to go back to his own house. Could I take him in my house? Certainly, it was the best solution, but we had to get him and carry him a long distance among armed Nazis patrols. The more dangerous moment would be the crossing of the bridge from the northern sector of the city where he was, to the southern sector of Rome where I lived. The two sisters, the mother, and myself, we could transport him with the help of some strong blankets and ropes. We planned the details and decided to meet in a certain place in the northern part of Rome.

I calculated that the trip back and forth would take me two days because of the long distance that we had to go in order to find my friend. Due to the curfew, we could walk only during full day. There was no time to think too much. The war situation was very unstable. The Allies could arrive at any moment and the Nazis would probably blow up the bridge that we had to cross. The conditions of my friend were deteriorating every hour. He had been drinking the contaminated water of the river with severe consequences for his health. I had to go and help. Would I tell my mother or Adeline? I decided not to.

I left quietly at sunrise after writing a little note saying that I would be back by the evening of the next day. It was a clear spring morning, blue skies, and a soft breeze. I walked fast. Running would have been suspicious. I avoided the main roads and took shortcuts to reach what used to be the central train station. The place was deserted, only a Nazi military truck was guarding the premises. I headed toward the central park, Villa Borghese. It had become a camping ground for all kind of people, mostly black market dealers. It was highly dangerous, but it was the shortest route.

Hurrying across the park, I remembered when, as a very young teenager, I had been horse riding in the park on Sundays among other young people. We were happy and looking forward to a brilliant future. Now, most of my friends were dead. Margaret died at sixteen of tetanus; Louise at seventeen of pulmonary tuberculosis; Ann, my best friend, was blown up by a bomb in a train when she tried to escape from the city with her family; Gregory was shot dead on the spot by a Nazi patrol. All were obscure victims of the war, of the lack of medical treatment and of the general disaster that had overcome a flourishing nation that was Italy before the war.

I run most of the time when crossing the park. The sun was high in the sky when I reached the stairs going down to Piazza del Popolo. I rushed down and there was the large empty Piazza with its beautiful fountain in front of me. I had to cross that vast solitary space to reach the bridge on the river Tiber, but I did not dare to walk cross the Piazza in the open. So I walked all around it, merging with the buildings, until I reached the bridge.

Nazis patrols were on both sides of the long, wide bridge. I swallowed my fears and walked as normal as I could. It was not possible to hide anywhere, as the bridge was a wide-open space and no one else was crossing it at that moment. I was in full view and easy to capture, but the soldiers were probably worried about their own situation. I safely reached the other shore and quickly disappeared into side roads.

Shortly after reaching the northern side of the river, I met the other three women, the two sisters, and the mother of my friend. They had the blankets, the ropes, and some water for me. I really needed the water.

During the occupation it was considered a crime to be in a group of more than three people, so we split in two groups of two walking at a good distance from each other. We headed to the house of the little girl who had discovered my friend. We would spend the night there. Entering that house took us a long, long time. First, the mother went in. The three of us continued walking in different directions. The younger sister was to be the second entering the house, but a patrol was too close and she did not dare to go in. She continued to walk straight and we lost sight of her. The older sister decided to try her luck and went in. No one noticed. I could not keep standing there and watching that door. I took a long walk, hoping that the patrol would go away. I was very tired and the sun was almost setting, when I finally came close to the house again. No one was around and I went in. I found that everybody was inside already. We had a simple soup and a good night sleep on the floor.

At dawn we left, one at a time, the little girl guiding us. The return to my house had to be a one-day trip, so we had to hurry. We found my friend, but we had no time to talk. He looked very sick and avidly drank the water that his mother had brought. We prepared the blankets and the ropes. Two long ropes, one on each side, were to be carried by four people. A third rope was linking the two main ropes horizontally in four spots, like an "S." In this way, a human body could be supported, if lying straight in the middle. We put the blankets on top of the ropes and my friend inside the blankets. We told him to lie straight and not to move. Fortunately, it was a deserted place protected by shrubs on the riverbank and nobody was around watching. Each one of us grabbed one end of the two main ropes and one corner of the main blanket. We folded the other blanket on top of him and we started our trip back.

If a military patrol would stop us and ask questions, we were lost. Maybe we could say that the man was dead, but you cannot be very convincing when you must say a lie in German. Anyhow, we hoped that they would imagine that we were carrying a dead body. That was not a rare occurrence. There was no other way of getting rid of dead bodies, but to carry them. There were no cars available, nor public transportation of any kind. We hoped for the best. Our goal was to reach the park by midday. The poor man was not heavy; he was almost a bag of bones. The mother had some food and water for him and we had a great hope to save his life.

Before reaching the crossing of the bridge, we stopped. There were some women carrying water buckets and we begged for some water. We pretended that the man was dead and we asked about the war. They gave us alarming news. The Allies were closing in and the bridges would be blown up as soon as the Nazi rearguard had crossed it; maybe today, maybe tomorrow, or, who know? We had to hurry. We headed south for the bridge among large groups of soldiers going in the opposite direction, but we found no patrol. No one paid attention to us; they were worried for themselves. We were safe!

Once we reached the park, we stopped again; a decision had to be taken. Only the older sister would continue to my house. My friend had to find the strength of walking supported by the two of us. The mother and the younger sister would go back to their house immediately because, if we were cut off and the bridges were blown up, there was no possibility of supporting four people at my place for several days. By then, we had only a few hour of the day to reach my house, or we would run the risk of being shot for not respecting the curfew. It was a though walk, but we calculated that we could make it. So, the two women, the mother and the younger sister, went back to their house and the three of us started on our long and slow walk toward my house.

I still don't know how we made it before curfew, but when you are really desperate you can do unbelievable accomplishments without even thinking about the circumstances. My mother was extremely upset when I arrived home with a sick man and a woman. She was right, but what else could I do? We took great care of my friend and he survived the ordeal.

The bridges over the Tiber were never blown up. The Allies entered in Rome June 5, 1944. We had been almost at the centre of the battlefield since they first landed in Sicily July 19, 1943.

Finally, the bloody war ended in May 1945.

The official dead toll was of about fifty two million people and the entire European continent was in ruin.

When we all felt that the war was over, in August 1945 came the horrible surprise of the atomic bomb on Hiroshima and Nagasaki. That was the most awful attack to a civilian population in the history of humanity. Half a million of innocent city dwellers were incinerated instantly and the following generations continued to suffer from radiation effects. The atomic bombs were totally unnecessary because the war was over. I remember very well and I was there.

It was ridiculous to pretend that Japan alone could be a dangerous enemy at that time. Japan was barely surviving after all the destruction and bombing.

The profound emotional wound that the horrors of war opened in my teenage years remained deep and painful for many decades. It took me many years of struggle to finally find the Master that was able to heal the wounds of my traumatic stress disorder. At last, he restored my emotional balance and my faith in a Benevolent Cosmic Power.

During the war, times and times again, I had addressed the cherished image of Jesus the Sheppard, remembering the white marble statue that I had contemplated in the Nun's chapel as a young child. I could not believe that a Loving God could exist and permit such brutal carnage. It must have been a cruel lie, just a story for children invented by the Nuns; the reality of war and destruction was too powerful and overwhelming, and I could not believe in goodness and in trust. For many years I was separated from the Source of Love and just submerged in work and duties.

Getting out of Italy

The nightmare of World War II was over and I wanted to get out of Europe. My dream was to open my wings and fly away!

I was thinking that somewhere in the world there should be peaceful happy people … that there should be open prairies, green hills, beautiful seashore, rivers and lakes without mine fields and bombs … that there should be strong, healthy horses to ride in the wind … I wanted to find a place to be free!

I wanted to go away from Europe.

I was twenty years old and full of life, but I could not leave my mother alone. I had to find a husband for her. When you really want something, then you find solutions. I put an ad in the local press.

"Healthy, middle-aged lady, retired teacher, economically independent, seeks gentleman similar conditions for serious relation. Please send hand written introduction of yourself."

I got many answers. A quick examination of the content, grammar, syntax, and handwritings, with the help of some knowledge of graphology, made me discard several of the letters.

I selected three letters and decided to talk with my mother. It was time for her to get out of her depression. She was surprised. We had a good laugh together and then I went into the task of contacting the senders. I met all three of them, but discarded two of them.

The winner was a retired lawyer, tall, gentle, intelligent and with an acute sense of humour. I liked him. He became eventually my stepfather; the new marriage of my mother lasted happily for more than twenty five years, when she became a widow for the second time.

I also traveled by train across Italy trying to find if some of our relatives in the north had survived the war. Taking a quick trip to Siena and Florence, I contacted local people about my father's relatives, but none was alive. The same thing happened with my mother's relatives in Verona and Padova in the north. I came back to let my mother know the sad news than no one in our close family had survived the war. Only the neighbours remembered some of them. Too bad!

Somehow, I felt that my mother was right to be so depressed. She and I were alone in the world with no relatives or family to support us.

By the time all this happened I obtained my passport and I had chosen Venezuela in South America as my dream country.

During the post-war time several countries in Africa and in South America were open to Italian immigrants. I faced a difficult choice among so many possibilities. I did a careful research in the Central Library and found that Venezuela had the most extraordinary natural beauties. Besides, it had a great potential as oil and iron producer and exporter. Venezuela was also rich in agriculture, in forests and in minerals. It had a long coast on the Caribbean Sea in the north and a rugged mountain range with high snow covered peaks running from north to south toward the west. The Great Plains and the large Orinoco River were toward the east of the country. Finally, unexplored Amazonian forests were occupying the south at the border with Brazil.

It was a dreamland! The land for me! So, I applied and obtained my immigrant visa for Venezuela.

In the month of May of 1947, at age twenty-one, I finally sailed away to my new life. Adeline, my mother, and my new stepfather remained in our house in Rome. I sold some apartments and the street shops of our building for my own expenses and left the rest of the apartments to my mother for her to live-in and have some income.

When the ship was ready to lift the ankles from the port of Geneva, it whistled a long final signal of good-by. At that moment I understood that something really important was happening in my life. I was abandoning my homeland and jumping into an unknown future. I looked around to be very aware of the moment and promised myself never to forget it.

I can still see the multitude on the docks waving white handkerchiefs (none of them for me), the very blue Italian skies, and the grey city with the mountains at the back. I said good-by more with a sense of accomplishment than with a nostalgic emotion. What I was doing was the right thing to do. I was not responsible for the misery and the destruction brought about by the bloody war. It was not my duty to stay at home to rebuild what senseless adults in search of power had ruined. I had suffered enough. I felt that it was my right to look for a new life in a fresh country. I was profoundly certain of doing the right thing and I never looked back on my decision.

Then, I started to explore the ship taking a walk on the deck; I found that its name was Lugano. It had three decks and I could walk freely almost everywhere. There was only the tourist class, so that all the ship was accessible. My cabin was for two people, as expected in all ships and I had chosen the bed on top, so I could look out from the small round window into the waves and the sky.

Talking later with the crew, I learned that the ship was a survivor of many past adventures and this voyage would be its last across the Atlantic. It would remain functioning along the coasts of Central America because it was too outdated for long trips. I felt that I was having a real adventure on a buccaneer ship! The rudder was not automatic and had to be held by a master helmsman. I was fascinated and spent long hours talking to the pilot and watching his skill. Once he finally let me hold the rudder and guide the ship. I was excited and happy, but the commander rushed into the cabin and kicked me out of my new adventure.

I saw other people being seasick, but I never felt anything. It was wonderful to have good regular meals, that I had missed for so many years and I just enjoyed myself with the wind and the sea. We crossed the strait of Gibraltar, the so-called column of Hercules, the end of the world for ancient sailors. The mountains of the coast of Africa were on our left side and the rocks of southern Spain on our right side. Our ship stopped at the Azores Isles and I experienced a great emotion buying sweet bananas from the local people and eating them walking on the docks until it was time to embark again. I had not tasted bananas for years!

During the trip I was supposed to learn Spanish. I had a beginners' book and intended to memorize some useful sentences, but I never did. It was much more important for me to enjoy the sun, the sea, the wind and to dream about my new life! The mood on board was not a happy one. We were all emigrants and most people were worried, sad, and silent. The captain tried to organize dances and parties, but people were not willing to laugh and have a good time. I stayed by myself, reading and relaxing.

After seventeen days of navigation we reached the coast of Venezuela. What scenery! Green hills and mountains all along the coast and little white, pink, yellow, and blue houses all along the slopes. My heart was beating fast with the emotion of looking at my new country. It was beautiful and friendly, prosperous and inviting. I was happy.

We disembarked in the port of La Guaira.

It was the end of a long struggle and a new future shining with hope.

Times of Peace:
My New Life in Venezuela (1947–85)

My new Country.

In my new country simple people living in a
Free, prosperous land were happy and friendly

Before landing, I did not realize that I was not prepared to face the different life stile that Venezuela and Caracas would offer me. The people were happy, free; they had plenty of food, social interactions, and entertainments. All this was too much, too new for me. While on the ship, the social environment was quite similar to the one I was used to in Italy. No one would talk too much, make jokes, be too happy, or laugh too loud. Our emotional wounds were still very fresh and the habit of silence and endurance were deeply established by the period of dictatorship and by the five years of war and military occupation.

The ship Lugano was the first immigrant ship to land in Venezuela in June of 1947. We were all young people running away from the horror of Europe and we were still mourning our own lost youth and our dead relatives.

On the contrary, for the people who greeted us in Venezuela, it was an occasion for much enthusiasm, joy, and happiness. The reporters came to the ship to take pictures and interview us all; on the next day, we were first page news on all the local newspapers. This expansive, joyful attitude of welcome of the whole population was great on their part, but let me confused and wondering what to do. Groups of us landed immigrants, were invited for lunch at different places, welcomed in private homes, treated as long-lost dear ones, and taken care of, as unique precious individuals. That was such an amazing display of friendliness, so much to eat, so much to enjoy, that I got dizzy. The cultural shock, the amount of food, the wonderful tropical fruits, and milkshakes were exquisite for my taste, but too much for my habits; the confusion with the language and the constant funny situation of using hands and body language to understand each other, were stressing my capacity to adjust.

After the first week I had to stay in bed alone and in silence in my hotel room for three days to be able to rest and recover. My energies had been completely drained. I know now that this happened because I am such an introverted person, but I did not know this aspect of myself at that time. Anyhow, I am very grateful still today for such a warm welcome to my new country. It allowed me to achieve a great jump in self-confidence and to start opening myself to the possibility of friendship. It was a sudden and tough awakening to a new life, but a welcomed one.

The natural beauties of the capital of Venezuela are unbelievable! A range of green, imposing high mountains separates the sea toward the north from the valley of Caracas. More toward the south, another range of gentle hills closes the whole scenery. The temperature is perfect, between 25 and 32 degrees Celsius during the day and a bit cooler at night. The wind from the northeast is refreshing and perfumed with tropical scent. The sky is intensely blue and vast. It is a dream place to live in. I was luck to be able to establish my residence in Caracas several years later. I lived there for a long time. Unfortunately, when I just arrived, it was too expensive for me to stay; I had to find another university in a smaller town.

At the Universidad de Los Andes in Mérida, Estado Mérida, I was accepted as a student in the third year of Medicine, as transferred from the university of Rome. I prepared to say goodbye to my new wonderful friends in Caracas. Before leaving, we did a special trip to the high mountains overlooking the coast. What an incredible view! From about four thousand feet, you can see on one side the vast expanse of the blue Caribbean Sea and on the other the green tropical city surrounded by luxuriant hills toward the south. I was so happy that I had to cry! My new country was so incredibly beautiful, generous, full of love that it was more than I could ever expect! I was overwhelmed with joy and gratitude!

A student and a hiker in Mérida and in the Andes' Range

To reach my new location in Mérida, I took the plain. Another incredible pleasant surprise expected me there.

In those days, the small city in the Andes was just a university town. It is located at about seven thousand feet, on a plateau facing immense snow peaked mountains toward the northeast. It is separated from this mountain range by a deep, large, canyon carved by an imposing river running south toward the plains. It is called Rio Chama. More mountain peaks surround the main plateau where the city is built.

A dirt road winded up toward the north to a mountain pass about twelve thousand feet high and another road connected the city with the plains toward the south. What a challenge for my longing for freedom and adventures! The view was spectacular from everywhere! Looking down from the airplane before landing I could imagine to be reaching Shangri-La, the valley of eternal youth.

When I disembarked at the airport, I found a large crowd. I could not imagine that so many people were traveling from such a small airport. Soon I found out that they were not passengers, but local residents enjoying themselves. As it was Sunday, the local custom consisted in going to the airport after Church to see who arrived from Caracas. Everybody in town was there, as if to greet me! Can you imagine my surprise? I received again a similar welcome as in the capital. It is unbelievable how friendly and cheerful are people who have not been harassed by violence and by war! I was invited for lunch at several private homes and just in a few days I had more friends interested in my welfare than I ever had in my entire life!

It was decided that the best for me was to live with the nuns. That society was very conservative and it was clear for them that a young lady like me should not live alone, but under the protection of an established institution. It was fine and it was cheep. My only duty was to be at home by nine pm and to go to the chapel for a Rosary at night. The nuns had a residence for schoolgirls and the place was neat and clean.

What a relaxing moment when I was able to unpack for good!

I had landed in an incredibly beautiful place and the people who surrounded me were the kindest I could ever think of! My little room suited me well. Just a bed with warm blankets and a desk with a chair for my studies. My two blouses and two skirts were hanging on a rope in a corner. That was all I had and all I needed to start my new life. I was incredibly happy!

The next day I went to the bank to open an account with the little money that I had to survive for the next four years of university. It was the product of selling some apartments of our house in Rome. I hoped to need less than two hundred Bolivares a month for board and food during four years; plus, university fees and books, stretching my scarce resources until the end of my studies. That was tough, but finally, I almost made it as planned.

The greatest concern was the language. My first written exam was due in October, little more than three months later. I had to become familiar with all the technical terms as fast as possible. I started to study very seriously Spanish and my new medical textbooks as soon as I arrived.

From that moment on, and for the next four years, I studied and studied and wrote tests; I presented exams, and took turns in the local hospital; I did not care about anything else. My mind was totally focused on graduating. I new that I was alone in the world. People, professors, and colleague students were very kind, but

I was aware that I could really count only on myself. I removed from my mind the memories of war.

Hard times were forgotten, Italy was forgotten, and just a few letters exchanged with my mother reminded me occasionally of my past.

The natives of the mountains and Herr Max

My only distraction from studying was hiking in the mountains on weekends, most of the times alone. I had only one friend, a university colleague, and a nice young lady, who was to be a close friend of mine in later years, but she was more involved with her fiancée than with a passion for hiking.

By wandering alone in those mountains I had the opportunity to get to know first hand the people of the Andes, the little farmers and the life of the poor at high altitudes. There I found real, sincere, simple, and honest human beings. They were serious hard workers, competent in their crafts, and extremely open and trustful. The children were the first who used to welcome me at the end of a steep path climbing up to some isolated groups of houses. They were round like little balls inside their heavy coats and caps. Their cheeks and lips were red because of the altitude and the cold wind. They looked healthy and were playful and trusting.

No cars, no machinery of any sort, polluted the fresh mountain air. The narrow paths reaching up to high slopes were good only for hiking or for donkeys carrying loads. Everyone looked in good shape because of so much exercise and pure air. Even very old, all wrinkled, men and women climbed and descended quickly those trails with steady feet. The farmed fields were ploughed with the help of oxen and were difficult to work because of the abundance of stones that had to be removed by hand every year. New stones surfaced from the dept of the earth at every season. The only entertainment of those peasants was the music provided by small radios and the occasional excitement of dancing in their yards in times of marriages or new babies.

The deep moral dimension of this peoples' culture was an unending surprise for me.

I was coming from the blood stained, so-called 'civilized' world, from the world of alienation, competition, distrust, cheating, lust for power, criminality and aggression. I was carrying myself a heavy load of guilt and uncertainty. Here, in these mountains, I found people grounded in their lands, in their traditions, in their common life of reciprocal help and sharing. They were a people with a natural deep spirituality that represented their true way of life.

Respect for each other was the fundamental rule in the family and in the community. The tasks of each member were naturally assigned by tradition and by needs. All adults would work in the land, growing crops and caring for animals. Children would participate in adults' activities with enthusiasm as true members of the community, according to their possibilities. I never saw a child beaten up, forced to do something, or harassed in any way. Women were strong and highly respected. Their opinions were freely expressed and taken in serious consideration, they ruled in everything related to family, children education, health, and common traditions. At group meetings, discussions consisted of few words, long silences, some further comments and the final agreement was not necessarily expressed in words, but in a silent consensus. No one ever raised the voice or tried to diminish the importance of other's concerns.

At the beginning of my interactions with the people of the mountain, I would ask questions such as:

"Why are you doing this in this way?"

They would look at me with a little smile and the answer was:

"Because this is how we like to do it." With an emphasis on "we like." The underlying meaning being that "this is how we chose to do it, by our own free will, and as a result of our experience."

For example, potatoes are always cooked in water with some milk. Why the milk? It took me some time to find out that a few potatoes were left cooking in the pail until they dissolved and then the whole thing was used to feed the pigs. While the milk gave a good taste to the potatoes that humans ate, the added cup of milk provided proteins for the pig.

Similarly, all the details of the art of cultivating and harvesting at that altitude were ruled by methods that were efficient and carefully established in their usefulness. Each little portion of soil was used with love and attention. Each plant of corn, potatoes or broad bean, was cared for individually, as a precious specimen. The judicious rotation of plantations prevented the invasion by parasites and the exhaustion of fertility. Periodically, parcels of soil were not cultivated. They were allowed to rest every so many years, producing grazing soil for animals. At the same time the droppings of herbivores would fertilize the land again, making it ready for the next cycle of cultivation.

Conversation was not used at all as a pastime. The only noisy and a bit dazzling social gathering would take place some times on Sunday, if there was a marked in some community or if there was some wedding. Then, the priest would come and do a formal religious service in some small chapel. That was the only opportunity to drink some beer, the men with the group of men and the women by themselves. The children were running around everywhere.

These people were grounded in their legacies and heritage, they were fully aware of belonging to the mountains, to the soil and stones, to the springs and fresh ponds. They trusted themselves and each other; they were strong and solid in their inner core and in their external expression.

What a lesson and what an example for me! I understood and appreciated the existence of a new dimension of humanity having a serious desire for a productive, simple, serene, honest, and peaceful way of life. They had a full consciousness of being different from the civilized world, but without antagonism or hatred for the dominating society ruling outside of their mountains.

It was rewarding and enlightening to visit them, absorb their strength, their peacefulness. They were the heirs of the native indigenous populations of these lands. The same ones that were killed and tortured and that were decimated by the European conquistadors. The same ones that were victims of the all-pervasive greed and violence that still two thousand years later dominates the so-called civilized world.

For the first time in my life, I realized that humans are fundamentally good if they are not crowded, harassed, and threatened. If people can count on the support of sound traditions, of a trusting community life, of sufficient food production and sufficient space for each to feel free, they show their essential goodness. Greed and violence are unthinkable and would not be tolerated by the strong community values.

It was for me a profound experience that lasted four years and that changed my perspective on humanity and on my own future.

I participated a few times in their dances and celebrations of marriages until I became part of a small family group composed by a young couple with two children and a grandmother.

On one occasion, while I was visiting my new friends and helping them getting their vegetables ready to be taken to the next day market, I learned something new.

"Are you taking these eggs to the market?" I asked Juan.

"No, he answered, these are for Ermak."

"What do you mean by ermak?" I asked.

"He is a friend, he calls himself Ermak, it must be his name, I don't know what it means," said Juan.

"Do you mean that this friend of yours is not from around here?"

"No, he says that he escaped from some place far away."

"When did he escape?"

"Oh, many years ago, I was a teenager when he arrived here."

"Where did he come from?"

"Oh, I don't know, some place with evil people and he escaped. He does not like to talk about it. But he has lots of books that he got from the university."

"That is interesting! Can I meet him?"

"I don't think so. He does not like to see people. Just my brother and me. He was a friend of my father, peace to his soul! Now, we bring him food and he always pays well. He has some sort of pension. My brother says that he saw pictures showing that he was a military in his country. But I don't know."

Juan turned around to take care of his sheep. He did not like to talk anymore.

I became very curious and determined to find out about someone called Ermak, reading lots of books and secluded in those mountains. I did not insist because I knew that Juan would not say anything more, but I kept thinking about it. On my way down to the city, suddenly, the word 'ermak' sounded like 'Herr Max' Ah! This was a German name! The mysterious hermit could be a former German officer running away from the Nazis' persecution. That made sense. Juan was about thirty years old and the stranger arrived to the mountains about ten or twelve years ago, around 1937. Interesting!

Only about six months later, I finally had the opportunity to visit Herr Max. Juan had asked permission for my visit and early a Saturday morning we climbed to the hermits' refuge. The path leading to it was steep and winding, but almost invisible among the wild grass and rocks. We reached a small hidden valley, about one square kilometre in size, protected from the prevailing winds by high peaks on the north-eastern side, but open toward the south to a spectacular view of the distant ranges.

The land was carefully cultivated in terraces, according to the ancient Incas fashion and in the far west corner, at the border of a huge precipice, a little stone house could be seen among large boulders. The perfect hiding place for a hermit! He was a tall, vigorous man in his early sixties, wearing a large straw hat and with a broad smile under his thick grey moustache. Immediately I felt positively impressed and very decided to get the best out of this encounter.

We took Juan's vegetables to the little kitchen and I noticed how the house was clean and well kept. A big picture of Herr Max in full military uniform was on a desk near the small window together with the picture of a lady and a child. My assumptions were probably correct, but it was not the moment to talk about the past. We were more interested in the present.

Herr Max took Juan and me for a tour of his valley. The first thing we saw was a large hand made pond were rainbow trout were cultivated. Max was very proud of it and it was his main source of proteins. To build the pond he redirected the waters from a source high in the mountain; he created a small waterfall to oxygen-ate the running water, and dug the pond. In order to seal the bottom and the sides of the pond, he compressed branches, stones, and some cement that Juan's donkey had carried up. The trout were feed twice daily with worms cultivated under large piles of compost near by. The same worms were so abundant that they were also used to feed a few chicken. These were enclosed in a little stone patio and contributed with eggs and meat to provide proteins for our friend. The cultivated terraces showed healthy beans, corn, green onions, some potatoes, and other local vegetables.

Juan's brother provided salt, rice, and petrol for the stove and for the lamp on a regular basis. Juan provided butter, eggs, and vegetables twice a month. The water was plenty and the air was clean! What a paradise!

After we completed the tour and admired the settings, we were invited to a rich vegetable soup and some 'perico' eggs. Well fed and stretching our legs under the table, the time came for some talking about intimacies. I asked about the lady in the picture. Yes, they were his wife and child that he had to abandon in Germany, in Bavaria, more exactly. The boy was now studying music at the conservatory in Paris. The lady had died under the bombs in France. Father and son planned to meet some day, somewhere, after the son finished his studies. But, Herr Max was certainly happy were he was in that mountain range and did not seem to be eager to change his residence. He had developed a very interesting philosophy that I came to understand later on.

That first visit was followed by several others when Juan was taking the monthly goods to Max house. We would spend the day there helping him with his many agricultural innovations, new terraces for cultivation, and a new stone patio for more chicken. Max's main occupation was his little farm, but he was also doing some translations for university professors interested in research and needing updates on German publications.

Little by little I learned about his point of view with respect of the Nazi tragedy and the war. He had a vast culture and was very influenced by some Eastern philosophies. He regularly practiced meditation and yoga and was very serene and benevolent. He seemed to have reached a balanced outlook on life with the understanding that all events, good or bad, are due to appear, persist for some time and gradually disappear by themselves because of universal natural laws.

He used to tell me:

> *"The real goal of your life should be to feel free to love, both people and the universe, after you have set yourself free from all attachments, from all duties, from all ties.*
>
> *First, you have to work your way out of the tangle of limitations that suffocate your life. This tangle is called "the hell of attachment."*

It consists on being dependent on others, who do not understand you, in your search for answers. We all go through such hell when we assume that other people or other things can give us happiness. We cling to them; we are slaves of family and social rules and impositions. We even submit to voluntary humiliations. We always hope that—this is the real thing-. We always imagine that the source of joy is there, outside there, we can almost reach it …, but, no, it escapes again. It is always somebody's fault, if we missed that promised happiness, that permanent solution to all our problems. It just happened because of -her-, or -his- fault, that all went wrong, but next time, it will be right. And so, we start all over again, only to be frustrated once more by our attachments. There is no end to it until we close our eyes for good. There is no way out of the hell of attachment until you understand that it is just hell, a hopeless labyrinth.

"You must be able to say "No!" to this and "No!" to that. After you said "No!" you must feel happy about your decision and never look back on it. Gradually you decide to detach yourself from everything and everybody until the moment when you start questioning your own life. That is an alarm point! What happens is that you tend to get stuck into the rejecting process and don't realize that 'rejecting' is also a form of attachment. You wake up and say:

"Ah, Ah! I arrived at the turning point!" What are the limits of rejection? This is critical. If you are unable to stop, you fall into nihilism, all sorts of negativities and make your life really confused and miserable. It is then clear that you jumped on the other side of hell, "the hell of total solitude," the wasteland of despair. You are forever alone with no motivation for living one minute longer.

If you can keep your mind clear at this point, then, you finally understand. There is one universal link to life, and that is universal love! Do you see the sun shining? It does not ask for your permission, it does not expect to be repaid; it just does its function and is fulfilled by it. Its function is to shine. What grows under its shining is none of its concerns. So, the question arises: what is the function of humans? What is my function? What is your natural function? This is a major philosophical question. You can spend many life times reading all what has been written about this topic and never arrive to any conclusion. So, don't read too much, but think. What makes humans unique on this planet? We have a biological body adapted to survive in the environment of the Earth. We are not very differ-

*ent from plants and animals. We need to breath, to eat, to sleep. We
move, we reproduce, and we defend our hunting ground.*

*We have five senses like all mammals, a stomach, bowels, legs,
eyes, ears, and nose. However, we have something unique. What is
it? Can you tell me what it is?"*

"Yes, I said, humans have evolved a unique part of the brain called neo-cortex.
We have a part of our brain that is able to speak and to understand the meaning of
words. We also have another part of our brain that is not where the speech centres
are. That part is dedicated to intuition, to understanding music, art, feelings, and
can grasp abstract thinking beyond words."

"Exactly, said Herr Max, that part of the brain is the important part, the one
that should be developed because it is able to experience universal Love!"

"So, he continued, if I ask you the question again: What is the function of
humans? The answer is: To shine with their unique light, the light of their universal Love! It does not matter 'what for'. It is just the natural human task because
it is a unique gift from nature. When the natural task is fulfilled there comes
a natural happiness, a contentment that consists in being in harmony with the
universal law. We achieve a sense of order, stability in emotions, in purpose, in
achievements. Do you understand?"

"Yes, I see what you mean, but how do you achieve this condition?"

"By being independent, said Herr Max, by setting yourself free, by relinquish-
ing all kind of personal, petty attachments, but keeping the understanding that
you are a creature of the Universe. That for a certain period of time you are supposed to shine in love and beauty, just the same as a flower, as a mountain under
the snow, as a bird high in the sky. There is no 'what for', there is just 'to be'.

Remember:

> *"All things are as they are because in no other way can they BE".*
> *"Everything is connected to everything else, but everything is unique
> in its beauty and in its function."*

"This is the great lesson that you learn when you become free, when you
become your real 'individual' self and forget about the limited obligations of your
'personal' petty, little ego."

I repeated:
"All things are as they are because in no other way can they BE".

That concept was not easy to grasp; I needed time. I kept repeating:

"All things are as they are because in no other way can they BE".

"All things are interdependent, continued Max, your love and your shining will bring about a change in the universe. You will never see it, you don't need to know about it, but you have accomplished your function. You have transformed the potatoes you ate, the energy of biological life, into transcendent thinking, into "Unconditional Love"! Into accomplishment, joy, fulfillment, serenity, and finally, if you want to believe in it, into Eternal Spirit! Into Universal Mind!"

Then he asked: "Is all this too much for you to imagine?"

"Yes, I said, it is too much for the moment. I will write it down and we shell talk about all this a bit more. I need to think it over."

But, Herr Max decided that he wanted to instruct me more. A few days later he wrote a few considerations for me to read and think about. This was very kind of him and I still have those pages with me. I hope he does not mind if I report his writings here:

"What can I say to change your sorrow into serenity?"

Acting and thinking as a victim of superior powers makes the common person a true victim in his imagination.
A powerless victim, separated from the source of life and from true happiness.
A trash in the merciless winds and storms of destiny.
Suffering is overcome only by the practice of consciousness expansion.
By the practice of introverted and extroverted contemplation.
By rising to the recognition of one's own supreme subjectivity.
If you understand that you are the Subject, the world of Objects has no power over you.
Because the common person fails to merge into the expansion of this recognition process, because he persistently ignores his condition as The Subject, he is constantly dragged down by incidental, secondary details, by surrounding Objects, in the form of thoughts, people and events, that are viewed as binding.
He is enslaved by meaningless circumstances.
He gets identified with useless tasks often perceived as unpleasant.

He is oppressed by a constant urgent sense of duty, as if one's obligation would be to change and possess everybody, everything, and the universe.

The personal ego of this common person is so insecure and in such great fear of being useless, that it makes all sort of efforts to be considered important, needed and to influence society.

This empty effort causes lots of suffering, stress, and frustration.

The moment one starts the practice of consciousness expansion, the whole perspective of life changes and is released of heavy loads.

One Self is the only Subject.

The surrounding world of thoughts, nature, and society are the many Objects.

By simple grammatical and syntactic laws of speech, we know that the Subject is the actor and what counts in every circumstance.

Where the Subject rules, the Objects have no power of their own.

Why be slave of so many ups and downs?

Why being harassed by so many emotions?

Why drown into so many likes and dislikes?

Why persist in a painful identification with Objects?

Attachment to other people and objects plunges the common person into constant fights.

Identification with another person is painful because each Subject is different from another Subject.

But the power of desperate attachment forces the common human to struggle constantly to change in his own direction the life of the other subject, which is impossible!

The conflict goes on and on because the attachment reinforces the binding ties demanding strenuous attention and all vital energies.

When finally the common person realizes that the battle is lost, he feels drained, frustrated, and victimized.

And the same process repeats itself with more and more people because attachment is the fear of facing one self, until life energy fades.

One's life is completely wasted by confronting what cannot be conquered.

One should dedicate energy and attention to one's own consciousness as the Subject.

One should try to get to know the Subject.

Understand, cherish, love, the Subject.

A tiny dot is the Subject in each one of us.

It is a pure point of potential energy.

It has no dimension, no weight, but is the source of Being.
Remember that the atomic bomb, with all its destructive power, is
less than a handful of material.
Real energy, real essence does not need physical attributes.
The real Subject is the virtual point where the vortex of manifestation and the vortex of dissolution meet in a dynamic, pulsating encounter.
That is your unique You, the Subject, the universal I AM, the Self of All.
A Point of infinite, eternal potential.
The only bliss, serenity, happiness!"

I was very impressed by Herr Max, and by his words. I wrote all I could remember and understand of our conversations as soon as I went to my room.

But then, I had to study, prepare exams, and face the permanent fact that I was extremely poor and really alone on this planet. I was not emotionally in a wasteland; I was simply alone, with nobody I could depend on. I was not attached to my studies, but I was interested in them and I absolutely needed to start working as soon as possible.

Maybe philosophers were people with some kind of rent, or somebody feeding them. I should think about all this later. Nevertheless, I took note and remembered.

Much later, I understood the dept of Herr Max advices!

It took me years of reflection and meditation to fully grasp his wisdom!

Another episode that touched me deeply occurred one day on the mountains. I loved to wander on those peaks and slopes. There were solitude and peace, the wind in the valleys and in the peaks, the fog, and the strength of nature untamed.

One day I went walking alone far away from the village and from the houses. I climbed to a peak and sat on a stone admiring the imposing landscape. A ravine plunged into a narrow valley a few feet from where I was resting. In front of me, on the other side of the canyon, I could see huge peaks and mountain ranges barren of trees, but decorated by large rocks with fantastic shapes, in memory of the telluric crashes that formed the Andes. The scenery was powerful, primitive, and majestic. The sun was shining and the wind of these heights was blowing strongly filling my ears with its song. I lied down and merged with the mountain, with the grass and with the stones.

"What are you doing here?" I asked myself,

"Who are you, after all, and why are you here?"

Thinking and dreaming I fell asleep, a restful, invigorating, profound sleep, but when I woke up it was getting dark and the evening fog was quickly coming up from the valley.

The fog in these tropical mountains is thick with humidity, dense and impenetrable, there was no way that I could find the return path down the slope. So I got up, found a niche under a large stone, put up the hood of my coat and sat comfortably leaning against the rock. For some time I watched the night set in and the fog raise from the depth. Then, suddenly, I was completely into the fog. I could hardly see my own hands. This is when you feel really alone, cut off from everything, alone with God, if you are able to contact Him.

I felt like the primordial human being on earth. I felt like Adam, like Abraham, like Moses on the mountain. I rested my head on my bended knees, I embraced my legs to keep some feeling of warmth, and I started talking with God.

"Tell me God, why the war? Why the hatred? Why the wounded and the suffering? Why these huge mountains? Why the immense ocean that I crossed? Why these wonderful, strange people, simple and serene as living in another plane of existence? Why God, why everything? And, what am I doing here? If you put me here, now, you must tell me what to do, what to say, how to act. I don't know, I know less than Adam knew, I am as lost a Moses was. Who am I? What am I?"

A long time passed or just a few minutes, I don't know, but I had the feeling that God promised an answer for some time later. I had the feeling of some presence, of some reassuring comforting presence even if no direct answer was forthcoming. I felt peaceful, trusting and I may have slept, I don't know. When I raised my head and opened my eyes, a wonderful sight! A clear blue night, a star lighten sky and a bright moon illuminating the landscape! I could clearly see the path down the slope as a friendly moon was smiling above me! A song of gratitude and of joy broke out of my lips and happily I started my way down to the village and from there to the road toward the city.

That experience, that promise, stayed with me for ever. I knew that I had received the assurance of getting an answer to my questions when the time would be ripe. Now, I just had to do whatever I had to do, and don't ask too many questions. My task was to graduate, work, be useful and shut up! So, down I went, to the city, to my little room and back to my studies.

My first job: Rural Doctor among primitive tribes

After four years of hard work, July 21, 1951, graduation time came and my money was finished. I did not have a cent to pay for graduation fees. Fortunately, a benevolent professor agreed to lend me about a thousand dollars from his own pocket to help me with graduation expenses and to get a job.

After the formal graduation, I was able to pay for a trip to the capital to sign my two years contract with the Venezuelan Ministry of Health, as a rural doctor in the State of Zulia. Once I had a working contract, I got a car, a 1950 Chevrolet.

I sent a message to Adeline to get on a plane and join me as soon as possible. I packed my few stuff and, driving toward the low lands of the west of Venezuela, toward the Lake of Maracaibo, I faced my future commitment.

In Caracas, when I signed my contract with the Ministry of Health, I was told that, before going to my assigned location, I should have a meeting with the chief of police of the main department. When I arrived in Marcaibo, the capital of the State Zulia, I went to see the chief of police and he told me:

"So, you are going to be the doctor in the Urdaneta district? I cannot let you go there alone and unarmed! What do you want, a gun, a rifle, a pistol or a revolver?"

I was shocked: "What?" I said, "I hate those thing! I left my country because of the war and I hate all weapons."

"You need to be armed, he said, because of the smugglers, they may be dangerous!"

"Ok, I said, give me the small stuff."

He gave me a pistol and a revolver. I did not know the difference, but on the spot they showed me how to use and clean them. They also gave me bullets and extra small bullets to practice shouting. I must say that later-on I practiced and became a very good gun-lady!

That same day, with my two guns and my personal belongings, some water and food, I started the trip toward the coast to go to *La Ensenada, Estado Zulia, Distrito Urdaneta* my residence village. The paved road ended at certain point and I drove for about 70 Km in a trail of deep sand. Driving in a sand trail is like driving in fresh snow. You have to keep in the tracks and go as fast as you can. Don't touch the brakes and don't think on turning around, because you can't. You have two walls of soft sand on each side. So, just go!

Finally, the path opened up and I came to the main village. What a surprise! A beautiful blue, large lake, a soft sandy beach, coconuts palms everywhere, and all the people around in the village doing their chores. Everybody was there, children, old people, donkeys, chicken, pigs, goats, women, and men. The whole population working, singing, playing under large straw roofs for protection from the sun. They were very friendly and happy to meet me.

They took me to the doctors' house. It was a very comfortable large house on the lakeshore with a private beech. It had been build especially for the very hot climate of that place. The lateral walls were about two meters high. On top there was an open space, between the walls and the roof. There the breeze could blow through, so that the house stayed relatively fresh and the air circulation was ensured.

Next, we visited the hospital. The small construction was built in the same way. It had two rooms for hospitalization of emergencies, a surgical room, an office/examining room, a large waiting room, and a lab space with no equipment, but proudly occupied by the only refrigerator available in the village. It was a very old one, working on petrol and requiring close vigilance.

The village had no electricity, no telephone, no running water; none of those things that we consider granted. I learned later that the water for daily use in the village was collected from the Lake of Maracaibo every day at dawn and that electricity could be obtained by motor plants, when they were repaired and working, but would be shut off at 10 p.m. anyhow. Fortunately, shortly after my arrival we started to have running water for the hospital and for the school, brought in by pipes from the oil fields in San Francisco, a nearby district.

The two ladies who were the assigned hospital keeper introduced themselves on occasion of my first visit and I was very happy to get to know my main helpers. They were Carmen, the mother and Rosa, the daughter. Carmen was an active, small and bony woman with an incredible sense of humour and the ability of smoking with the lighten end of the cigarette inside her mouth. I was astonished of this, but she would say that she did not want to drop the ashes of her cigarette on top of my desk or on the surgical instruments. Rosa told me not to worry because she had seen her mother smoke like this during all her life and it was unlikely that she would change her habits.

Rosa was in her twenty's and a very intelligent girl. She was taking correspondence courses to become a bookkeeper and an accountant. This was an exceptional effort and showed great determination in that environment of mostly illiterate people. She became quickly my assistant, nurse, and everything I needed. I knew that she was very responsible. This two women team was taking care of the hospital, cleaning it, keeping it in order, updating the books and stock of the pharmacy, and caring for the precious refrigerator where all the emergency drugs against snake bite, tetanus, rabies and all the vaccination were kept.

After the excitement of the trip, the arrival, and the meetings, I was exhausted, but I had no bed to sleep in. I asked if someone had a new hammock for sale and fortunately, yes, it was found and I was able to settle in my house and sink into a profound sleep.

In the following days I met the police officer, the chief of the village, the schoolteacher, and the main citizen. I was taken with the police car (the only transportation available, beside my own car) to visit the other two villages under my jurisdiction, El Carmelo and Palmarito. I soon realized that I was going to face a lot of work, long distances and a rural population spread out among sandy dunes between the lake shore on one side and the deep jungle on the other. But, I also realized that the people were wonderful, friendly, open and expecting everything from me as from a goddess. The challenge was incredible and very appealing. They showed so much trust in me that I could not do anything else, but my best for them.

There had been no doctor in that area for the last two years, so everything needed a fresh organization. I asked for everybody's help. We had a first meeting and different activities were organized. The school children needed special attention as they all had lice in the hair and intestinal parasites. The teachers and a couple of mothers would take care of that under my direction. I had inspected the jail and found it in bad conditions, so I closed it until it would be repaired. The police officer took care of that. The only tavern and restaurant needed sanitary improvements, so I closed it, and the chief of the village would take care of that. I inspected several septic tanks in private houses and found that some were full and overflowing menacing to contaminate the water of the lake. A commission of citizen took care of digging new sanitary tanks and repairing others according to rules. After the first week, I could finally start being a real doctor and doing consultations.

Adeline arrived shortly after. She had an adventurous trip by plane from Rome to Caracas and then traveled during four days by bus without knowing a word of Spanish. She was a thought woman and survived!

The first problem I met being a real doctor was my lack of expertise. How easy it had been practicing in the hospital where lab reports were available x-rays quickly done and other colleagues could be consulted in case of doubt. Now, I was alone, no lab work possible, no x-rays, no colleagues, and a lot of new unpredictable emergencies.

For a diagnosis, I depended exclusively from my five senses and from my skill. I quickly learned to recognize certain smells. Fever, diarrhoea, bronchitis, urinary problems, and others, all smell in a different, characteristic way. The touch of my hands on the skin of the patient would tell me a more precise story. The sound of heart, lungs, bowels, would add more information. Finally, my eyes would confirm or change the total diagnosis. I never learned so much in medical school, as I was forced to acquire in a few weeks as rural doctor.

The "fever"

One of my first serious patients was a night-call because of "the" fever.

I did not know that the name "the" fiver, meant, malaria. I expected to see a boy running a temperature, maybe a cold, but when I arrived, I was shocked to see that the walls of the small hut were shaking. A young man in the hammock was shivering intensely, all his muscle tense, burning with fever, and almost unable to breathe.

This was my first case of serious malaria. I had a full pharmacy in my car, so I was able to inject the patient, take care of him, and I stayed until morning when he finally got better.

Sleepless nights like that first one became more and more frequent later on. At seven in the morning I was in the hospital attending the lined up patients until noon. Then, I would take a break and have a little sleep until three p.m. when the afternoon consultation would began until six pm. After a short break and supper, the home visits would start at eight p.m. and continue during the night as needed. Fortunately, I was young, enthusiastic, and strong, but the work was exhausting. The satisfactions were many.

The diabetic lady

One of the most dramatic cases was a middle-aged lady who was supposed to be dying of cancer of the uterus. The family asked me to see her because she was dying and they would need a medical certification of the cause of death. So, they thought that I should be informed and examine her before she died.

They had already prepared the house for the funerals. The bed of the patient was in the middle of the entrance room of a large, comfortable, almost rich house. A layer of fresh sand had been put all around the bed, as custom for funerals. Relatives were arriving from everywhere, as the lady was an important member of the community. The patient was unconscious and partially covered by an elegant blanket. Only the funeral candles were missing.

As I went in, a characteristic smell hit my nose. I perceived a strong smell of rotten apples. It is described in all textbooks as characteristic of diabetic coma and acidosis. My mind raced, this woman was dying of high blood sugar. I would not let her die. I still could do something. Without the help of lab controls, I risked using intravenous insulin; it was a desperate fight between death and me. I stayed at her bedside for almost ten hours, slowly controlling the vital signs and the effects of insulin, fluids, and electrolytes replacement therapy. I had intravenous glucose ready, just in case. It became a slow struggle that lasted hours, given the risk of a sudden death. But miraculously she emerged from the coma and opened her eyes. Unbelievable, she would not die for the moment!

The relatives could not understand what was going on, but finally, after the firsts few hours, I was relaxed enough to start talking with them. The diagnosis of cancer of the uterus was made erroneously based on some vaginal discharge that the patient had, probably due to a fungal infection that is frequent in diabetes. Nobody had ever suggested that she was a diabetic, so she went into coma because of very high blood sugar and acidosis.

Later, this patient recovered fully and two years afterward she was an active member of her community, happy and with her diabetes well controlled. This case was a great satisfaction for me.

The enlarged prostate

Another dramatic case was a middle-aged man who could not pass urine and refused to be taken to the hospital. He insisted that he wanted to die in his home and his mind was clear and strong, so, nobody could force him. The relatives called me because he was going to die of urinary retention and I had to certify the cause of death. They did not expect that anything could be done at home because they had been told that the patient needed a supra-pubic incision and a catheter inserted in the bladder. This procedure could only take place in a hospital.

I went to see the man. He was angry with everybody and only wanted to die in peace. So, we started a conversation. I could see his full bladder, like a big ball, in the lower part of his abdomen. Obviously it was a case of severe prostate enlargement that prevented the flow of urine from the bladder. Patiently, I suggested that he let me try to insert a catheter.

"I will do what is possible without hurting you, I told him, I may fail, but lets try, if you are willing to cooperate."

Finally, he did agree.

From my large bag I took out a series of catheters of different sizes and a Foley. I prepared the field with sterile towels, put on my gloves, and started the procedure. Very slowly in deep concentration, I introduced in his penis a mid sized catheter, just to start, knowing that it would not go through. I needed that the patient relaxed completely, so I waited, using larger catheters at the beginning.

When I sensed that he was relaxing, I picked up a very thin catheter that was dangerous because it could create a false route. It could enter the soft tissues and cause an open wound that would become infected. In order no to create a false route I had to find my way in the narrow path of his enlarged prostate without creating a wound with the fine instrument. The pressure of my hand had to be firm but gentle, letting the urinary conduct guide the instrument. I told him that the procedure would be long, that I wanted him to relax and breathe slowly and go to sleep if possible.

We waited, and at a certain moment I felt as if the catheter had moved a few millimetres by it self. That was the indication that I was in the right place. I waited longer, with a gentle pressure. Again, the instrument progressed a few millimetres. After a certain time, I became confident that I was in the correct place, I continued the gentle pressure and was very alert and concentrated. Finally, I felt that some resistance had given way, which was a dangerous sign; did I create a false way? My heart started to beat faster, but the catheter went in and surprisingly, a flow of urine emerged.

We had won the first stage of the battle! The man could not believe his eyes looking at his urine coming out. We called in the wife and she started screaming with joy.

It took a long time until the bladder emptied through the small instrument and then we started the process of dilatation with larger catheters to be able to install a permanent Foley. The whole procedure took hours, but I left the man happy, with life and with a permanent catheter inserted.

Later, he accepted to go to the hospital and have his prostate removed and a proper procedure performed.

The Matriarchal Society

Cases like these gave me great satisfaction, but the pace of work was very demanding. Adeline was of great help. She had adapted quickly to the hot climate, to the simple people and to the use of petrol to cook. We had plenty of fresh food. Every day, from the shores of the village, several rowing boats would go fishing in the lake before dawn and a great variety of fish could be purchased on the beach early in the morning, when the boats came back loaded. We would get gifts of fresh eggs and of tropical fruits such as bananas, coconuts, and pineapple, from grateful patients and we needed to purchase just rice, salt, and a few other items from commercial stores.

The local people were descendent of the Caribbean tribes of warriors and navigators. They called themselves Goajiros and followed a matriarchal tradition.

What is a matriarchal community? It is a community ruled mostly by women, by old women who have been trained to lead and who remember everything about traditions, medicine, and social rules. They are living archives of the history of every person, of how to do every task, when to fish, when to hunt, who should mate with whom, who is related to and should not have children with, all the details of the history of past and present generations.

Their authority derives from their age and from a real knowledge that is essential for the social functioning. Each village is a clan run by the oldest woman of the community. In each clan there are families of women, each run by the oldest woman of the family. Each family has a space, for small houses, for animals and for children to play. Only old men or sick men can live in these houses, to be taken care of.

In the matriarchal society of those villages, at the time when I lived with them, every activity and every person would go through precise and well defined cycles. Young healthy males left the main women's house as young teenagers, became hunters, fishermen, and cultivators, and did all the outside tasks by turn. At certain age, they mated with the assigned young girl. They build their provisional hut and took care of the woman and children until two of the children born from that union were able to walk. After a couple had two children that survived and walked, the girl returned to her family and would not mate again for a period of time.

This is how they kept birth control. The man continued to do his tasks for the community and after a prescribed period he would mate again with a girl of a different family. This union continued until two children could walk. The woman also would mate a second time with another man, according to social rules.

When people reached an age of thirty five or forty they would not mate again. The average life span, at that time in those villages, was about fifty years of age. Seniors would be assigned different tasks and responsibilities, according to their capacity. Most women had three or four living children. The children would have the family name of their own father and, as a second family name, the one of the mother.

There were many tasks to keep everybody busy all the time and they had many big social celebrations. It was a very simple and efficient life and I learned a lot from them. There was no money, everybody contributed somehow, and exchanges of goods and labour were the rule. There were no lies, because all lived together all the time, no greed because there were no personal possessions. The social discipline was very strict, but natural.

This experience showed to me again that humans are fundamentally orderly and peaceful if communities are properly organized and if there is respect, activity, and justice. People can function very well without any of the so-called modern commodities. What I learned stayed with me. I remember that there was happiness, joy of living, simplicity, and sincerity that transpired in all interactions among those people and I know that the true nature of humans is good!

Going fishing with the men

I got to know better my people during one night when I went fishing with them. For some time I had been interested in participating in a fishing expedition during the night, but the world of the fishermen was an entirely males world and no woman ever stepped into a boat.

My request was a matter of serious consideration and they would have denied my access to a boat if the patient that I saved from dying of urinary retention would not have spoken on my behalf. Finally, one day, one of the ladies who were matriarchal leaders sent a messenger to let me know that a propitious night had been chosen, if I was free and willing to participate in the night fishing.

Fortunately, that evening no one was seriously ill and I was able to be at the beach at the appointed time. Tree large boats left the shore in total silence, with five men each, four rowing and one at the helm. I was sitting in the middle seat in the boat of the chief. About a mile from shore, the rowing stopped in all the boats and the chief stood up and watched the skies in silence. I had the impression that he smelled the wind.

The moon was rising and the night was perfectly calm and full of stars. I cherished those moments of absolute tranquility and silence. After a long while the chief raised his right had in a certain direction, sat down and the rowing resumed very gentle, slow, and silent. We slid over the calm silvery water for a certain time and then the chief raised his hand signalling that we had reached the right spot for the night fishing.

The men got busy with the nets. The boats were aligned at the proper distance and we waited. In a very low voice I addressed the chief to thank him for allowing me to participate in that night fishing. He smiled and said: "Doctor, I don't know how to address a lady, as we are not used to have any one with us, but we are very grateful for what you are doing among us, so we decided to make an exception."

"I understand and I am also very grateful for your kindness. Now I would like to know, if you mind answering my question, what is it that you like the most about your fishing?"

He looked surprised. Probably he had never thought about such a question. Fishing was a natural thing that had to be done to feed the people, why was I asking about liking it?

To help him and make my question less aggressive, I asked him at what age he started fishing. He felt more comfortable with that concrete question and started telling me about his life. He was fourteen the first time that he faced a big storm and since then he had many other hardships, but he did not want to change his occupation and become a hunter or a worker. He liked the water, the wind, and the smell of the night. He continued to talk about his life as a fisherman until slowly the answer to my question came out by itself.

"You see, he said, each one of us has a special task, a special talent, a special way of being useful to our people. I found that I am good at finding where the fishes are. I understand the winds and somehow I know where fishes are feeding. So, this is what I do best, where I can be more useful, where I find satisfaction. The lake has been tough with me to teach me, but we have learned to get along. When I sit here in silence, I am able to listen to what my heart is telling me. The lake is talking to my heart, telling me what to do. I have also learned about the stars and how to find our way when there are no stars.

You need good companions because all depends on how everybody responds when there is a storm or a strong wind with high waves. They also understand the weather and the water as I do, so we trust each other. That is what our traditions say. We must learn to trust each other and to trust the lake. That is the reason we made an exception for you, because we have learned to trust you too."

When he spoke like this I almost cried with emotion and felt like embracing him. It was the most sincere expression of gratitude I ever received. To be trusted! What a great feeling! To live and work trusting each other, what a great way of living and working! You do what you do best to be useful to your people and you go along in life trusting each other! What a real goal in life!
No philosopher can match this true-life experience!

The night ended perfectly with a successful catch to feed the whole village and I had a new treasure in my heart, the awareness of being trusted!

More adventures at the lakeshore

During the first one and a half year that I was in that community, no smugglers bothered us, but one day when I was returning from a distant visit, something happened that was a bit stressful and that I still remember vividly.

One evening I received an urgent call from a family living far away in the dunes. The man who came to summon me had been walking for many hours to reach the hospital. He told me that there was a trail that could be used with the car to go very close to the patient house. When I enquired about who was sick he informed me that one of the old women of the clan had been having pain in her chest, fever and cough for some time, but recently she had been coughing blood, was very sick and could not eat.

I thought that it was probably an acute phase of long-standing pulmonary tuberculosis. So I gathered all the equipment that I would need, some water and food for my self, and my usual pistol and revolver, as we were going into the wilderness where smugglers used to operate.

By the time we left, night had fallen and it was pitch dark without moon. We followed the main car trail to the southern village of Palmarito and from there we continued south entering into smugglers country. There were lots of car trails in that wild area, as those people used large trucks to transport smuggled goods from the lakeshore, across the jungle, to the paved roads of the district. They smuggled mostly alcohol, cigarette, and weapons arriving by ship from USA and they paid with 'natural products', as I had been told. (Now I know that the so-called 'natural products' were cocaine leaves carried from the mountains, but I did not know this at that time).

The authorities had no funds to control the vast wilderness of the southern part of the lake and smugglers were all the time changing their routes and the sites of landing. So, the local police only cared that smugglers would not enter villages or do harm to local people. To catch them when they reached paved roads was the task of the interstate police. The jungle, swamps, and deserts were full of dangerous wild life, snakes, large carnivores, poisonous insects, and malaria carrying mosquitoes. Only smugglers would dear to transit through those places.

The man who had come as a messenger told me to take with me some strips of surgical gaze to tie on branches at crossing points of the trails in order not to get lost on my way back, as I would return alone. At each important crossing of trails he would step out of the car and tie a strip of white gaze for me to see clearly the return path. We finally reached the small houses on the far away side of the southern lakeshore.

I found the patient in bad conditions, almost terminal and beyond hope. My major concern was not so much about saving her life, as to isolate her from children and young adults. Open pulmonary tuberculosis is very contagious and my main task was to explain to that small community what to do, considering that they all were highly at risk. I scheduled appointments for all the children and young adults to be controlled for TB. I illustrated how to take care of the old woman needs wearing masks and gave other important instructions.

Explaining all these details took me a good part of the night.

Finally, I started my return home, hoping to be able to catch some sleep before the morning consultation. But, I was wrong! Suddenly, when I was already approaching the southern part of Palmarito a large truck stood in the middle of the path closing my way, with a running motor and high lights focused on me. I stopped, put on my high lights, and waited. There was no place where to turn or escape, large dunes of sand, cactus, shrubs, and desert all around.

"Here are the smugglers!" I thought "and who knows what they want." "They probably think that I am a competing smuggler and they are going to shoot. The best is that I don't talk, so that they don't find out that I am a woman alone."

Very slowly I grabbed my pistol and revolver from under my driving seat and moved over to the back seat for more protection. Very slowly I lowered the back window and I was decided to shoot if someone was coming toward me. Nothing moved. We stayed there watching each other for a long, long time. I was hoping that with daybreak they would leave. For me, every hour was an advantage.

Finally, the first clarity of dawn appeared on the east, over the lake. I knew that people from the village would be gathering water or walking on the beach. There would be groups on the shore not too far away.

That was my moment! I extended my right arm out of the window, started to shoot my pistol in the air, and yelled with all my lungs:

"Get out of my way, I am the doctor!"

To my great astonishment, a chorus of laughter responded to my screams.

"Oh! It is the doctor! Incredible! All this wasted time!"

Then, my friend the local chief of police appeared from behind the truck. There was already sufficient light and we could recognize each other clearly. What a release! But, my curiosity was now very great.

"What happened?"

Well, the story was that the police had seen the lights of a car going south early in the night (when I drove along the south shore toward the patients' house). They imagined that it was a new operation of the smugglers south of the Palmarito village and they had to stop it. So, during the night they called the police of the oil fields of San Francisco to help them with men and a large truck to stop the smugglers operation. They posted themselves at a key intersection and waited for the criminals.

Well, they caught me and we had a good laugh.

Other times, my duties were not so exciting, but always rewarding.

The missing finger

I remember one morning around five a.m., someone banging on my window and urging "Doctor, help me!" I got up and looked out of my window to answer that call for help, but I only saw the long hears of a grey donkey standing beside the house. I went out and found a man sitting on the ground and holding his left arm tight against his chest. In his right hand he was holding his left thumb. He was bleeding heavily and his shirt was soaked in blood. I got him quickly into the car to the hospital and with a few stitches I was able to stop the bleeding.

The story was that he was working early in the fields, cutting tall grass to feed his cow, when he cut his own left thumb together with the grass. He had chopped it completely off from the hand and the cut artery of the finger was bleeding profusely. Fortunately his donkey was nearby and by compressing the left hand under his right armpit he was able to reduce somehow the bleeding until he reached my house. He expected that I would sow his left thumb in place.

"Sorry, I told him, this has to be done in a big hospital. I don't have the equipment here. The chief of police will take you to the hospital as soon as possible."

The wounded man was worried thinking that he could not go to the city all soaked in blood, but I reassured him saying that in the emergency department, the more blood he had on himself, the faster they would take care of him. A few hours later the man was gone, carrying his cut finger in a bag kept cool in a container with ice.

Adeline took care of the nice grey donkey until someone came to pick it up.

I had forgotten about this case, when a few months later, on a Saturday morning, when I was preparing to go swim in the lake, the same grey donkey appeared at the gate of my house. On top of the donkey an elegant man, all dressed up for the visit, was smiling, and waiving both his hands with five fingers each.

"He got his finger plugged in!"

I thought, and invited him in to share his adventure. He told me that at the emergency they had attended him immediately, as I had predicted, and that the doctors had done a great job. I was very happy for him and for the successful outcome of a type of surgery that was still rarely effective in those years, due to the long time elapsed form the moment of the accident, the contamination of the wound, and the equipment of provincial hospitals. But, when there is good will and determination, events happen that look like miracles.

A miracle that did not happen

At other times, when I really wanted a true miracle, it did not happen.

It was about two in the afternoon, I was spending my midday "siesta" at the lakeshore in my hammock hanging between two palm trees and enjoying the breeze from the lake, when a vociferous group of people appeared at my gate. They came quickly in, carrying a body.

It was the body of a twelve years old girl who had drowned in a nearby beach. I rushed to the house and they laid the limp body of the girl on the floor of the sitting room. Immediately I started resuscitation procedures, but they did not give results. So, I decided to inject physiologic solution with traces of adrenaline directly in the heart. But nothing helped. The girl did not respond. She was gone from this world. We could not call her back. It was a sad experience.

The perception of death

I had several other sad experiences with elderly people having cardiac failures, with people with cancer, with patients with chronic malaria and mostly with children with acute gastroenteritis. But, the serenity with which the native people faced death taught me a different approach to mortality, as compared to the one that I had learned in the civilized world.

In a similar way as the people of the mountains, they had a natural, I would say dynamic, approach to life and death. Both life and death were inherent in reality and part of every-day awareness. For them, the ups and downs of human events were as obvious as sun rise and sun set.

There were no intellectual 'should' or 'could' between them and life. Females were supposed to raise children, males to feed them. When you have done your duty, you die happy and become a blessing presence for your relatives. When children die, they are considered angels, protectors of family and neighbours. When death comes, it is a traditional inevitability. They did not have our civilized arrogance pretending to fight against death. It was considered as absurd as stopping the sun from raising or from setting. So, I had patients who would decide that their time had come. They would refuse to eat and drink, turn the face against the wall and don't talk any more. Relatives would respect their decision.

I remember, at the very beginning of my practice in that village, the case of an old man with an advanced cancer of his lower lip due to cigarette smoking.

He was having intense neuralgic pain on his face because of the invasive tumour. I wanted him to go to the hospital in the city, receive treatment or surgery, do something, beside the sedation that I could provide for him. But, soon I found out that he had decided otherwise. When I went the next day, the daughter told me:

"Thank you for coming, but my father has turned his face to the wall."

That was it. Two days later he was gone. No one can survive in that climate without drinking. He had decided to stop suffering and the family respected his decision. No one would come up with rationalizations about the right or not of ending ones' sufferings. No one would discuss the old man self-euthanasia on cerebral considerations.

These are nonsensical objections of culturally-deviant-so-called-civilized people! Life and death are natural events that must be accepted as inevitable without undue resistance.

A tough decision

After a certain time of being a doctor in that community, I was often wondering what I would do next, when my two years contract with the Venezuelan government expired. I was only twenty seven years old and I felt like conquering the world! I could renew the contract for two more years, but it was unlikely. I wanted to specialize in some branch of medicine or surgery, but I had not made any choices, until one day I suddenly knew what I wanted to do.

It was a very tough decision involving much effort and dedication, but I decided to specialize in surgery and in gynaecology.

Mother and babies' care was one of the most important aspects of the hospital's activities. We had dedicated one of the emergency rooms only to hydration of babies presenting vomit and diarrhoea because of gastroenteritis.

My assistant Rosa was very skilled and responsible; her commitment spared me a lot of routine work. Nevertheless, the load of care for pregnant women was very heavy. I wanted to control personally all expecting mothers every month, but some times the line up was too long and some women would not stay on line to wait for their turn. So it happened that some of them developed water retention, albumin, and hypertension before delivery, because of lack of proper control. Most of the cases were mild and had no consequences.

Nevertheless, one special case run close to became a tragedy.

It was a very young girl in her first pregnancy. She was a friend of Rosa and also an exceptionally intelligent young woman. She incurred in severe water retention, kidney damage, and hypertension; in her last trimester, she suddenly developed convulsions. This is a life and brain threatening condition called 'eclampsy' due to the malfunction of the kidneys and hypertension.

One morning I received and urgent call from the family because she was having convulsions. I rushed at her bedside and started some emergency treatments, but after a few hours, she was not doing better. She was not in labour and both her life and the life of her baby were in serious danger. So, I decided to drive her in my car to the Maracaibo hospital. She needed an urgent caesarean section, or the baby would probably die and she could have permanent brain and kidney damage.

Under heavy sedation, we carried her to the back seat of my car where she could lie down while her mother would hold her head on her lap. I had to drive as fast as possible on those sand trails and then in the city traffic to the main hospital. It was hot, humid, and dusty, that trip was a nightmare!

The patient continued to be unconscious and to have occasional mild convulsions. Fortunately, the emergency department was not very busy and shortly after we arrived, we rushed her to the operating room.

I changed and washed at the same time as the resident doctor and assisted him during the caesarean section. My emotions were running high as I had much consideration for the patient. Finally, the baby was born and appeared to be healthy. It was a great first victory! Later, when the mother recovered from the anaesthesia, it became clear that she had not suffered brain damage.

I finally relaxed.

At that moment, I understood what I wanted to do for the rest of my life. I wanted to save mother's and babies' lives. I felt attracted to the supreme mystery related to the birth of a human being. I would become a gynaecologist. I wanted to take care of mothers and babies.

That was a final decision. It was a very tough decision.

I would go back to civilization, to university and specialize in Obstetrics and Gynaecology

I did not know at that time that the years that I spent as rural doctor would be the best memories of my early career. The simple life among those sincere people had restored my confidence and hopes in my own future. They loved me and I loved them. They needed me and I needed them. We enjoyed a constant frank, straightforward, brotherly interaction that healed my body and my spirit.

Everyday brought its own stress, its worries about some patient and then the release of tension, the solution of problems, when the patient got better. Emotional rewards constantly alternated with new responsibilities, but the play of tension and release was balanced by mutual trust and confidence. We new each other deeply enough and we were able to participate fully in good and bad moments.

I am profoundly grateful to those fishermen, hunters, and housewives, simple workers who gave me the gift of their unconditional trust. They put their lives in my inexperienced hands as they put their trust in God. I was the only intermediary who could help and miracles were trustfully expected. I look back to those times in wonder about the perfect relationship that developed between a young woman like myself, alone and harassed by life, and those native people emerging from past ages with their matriarchal society and primitive structure.

Probably we all felt so totally alienated from mainstream society, that it was rewarding to discover each other at the fringe of this modern world. The very essence of their freedom was constantly under the menace of progress and of the so-called civilization. My own independence had been temporarily saved only by physically running away from Europe. We were fugitives from the monster of politics, fanatics, indiscriminate authority, deep pervasive greed, and abuses. Somehow, without speaking we recognized each other, the spirit of ancient natives who fought against colonialism and the brutal invasion of their lands, and myself, a victim of the same cruelty and barbarism.

Post-Doctoral Studies in Europe and in Canada

When my contract expired, I left my paradise on the lakeshore, returned to the civilized world and during the next seven years, I specialized in clinical and surgical Gynaecology.

First in London, UK, at the Hammersmith Hospital, then in Milan, Italy, at the Clinic Mangiagalli and finally in Toronto, Canada, at Women's College Hospital and Toronto General Hospital. These years of specialization in different hospitals were very demanding to my health.

No time for private life, no time to exist as a person, just a dedicated, automatic "student" could survive the unending stress and the fast pace. Combining night shifts with classes, examinations, research, and papers-writing, was hard enough. On top of that, the extenuating duties of outpatients, operating room and emergency calls.

As all this would not be enough, we intern-doctors had to cope also with the hospital neurosis of professors, students, patients, and nurses. These conditions made the whole life a major struggle.

The seven years stretched my physical and mental resistance to the limits, but somehow I managed to accomplish all academic and hospital duties to the end. I became an accomplished specialist surgeon and clinician in gynaecology and the author of twenty-two scientific publications. In 1959, I obtained a Ph.D. in Italy, as the first woman to get such academic recognition in a surgical specialty.

In order to obtain my academic recognition as a contributing scientist, I dedicated a few years in Italy doing research on the Hystochemistry of cancerous cells at the University of Milan. That was in 1956-58, and the use of chemotherapy for the treatment of cancer was still at the experimental stage. My research on the biochemical characteristics of the cancerous cell in the field of Gynaecology, contributed to understanding the specific physiological metabolism of the cancerous cell of both the ovarian and the cervical cancer of the uterus. During the three years of research, I published 22 long articles with very technical data about the histology and chemistry of these cells that I observed at the microscope.

I also presented my works to medical congresses on Gynaecological Hystochemistry both in Italy and in France (as I speak French fluently). All my scientific research and publications were published during the late fifties, in the Italian "Rivista di Ginecologia."

Back to Venezuela

I completed my training as a Specialist in Gynaecology in 1960. I was thirty-five years old, a fully trained professional and ready to assume higher responsibilities. I could remain in Italy and become an assistant professor, or accept the position that I was offered at the university of Toronto, but the longing of my heart during all those years was Venezuela. It was my adopted country, I loved everything of it, the mountains, the coast, the sea, the people, the climate, the tropical flavour, the freedom of open spaces, and I remembered how happy I had been during my years as a student. I was still touched by the friendliness of the people who opened their hospitality to me when I first arrived as a lonely immigrant.

My love for Venezuela was profound and stable like the love for a dear person. I could not think on fixing my residence in any other country.

Therefore, I established myself in Caracas. I did not know anybody there, but in a short time, I got a position at the Universidad Central de Venezuela as professor of histology, and then I was appointed specialist doctor at the Maternity Hospital and assistant professor of Gynaecology. A brilliant academic career started, together with a rewarding private practice. Everything was going very well; I had achieved all my professional aspirations and only one aspect of my life needed to be fulfilled. I wanted to have children.

I had chosen my profession because of my appreciation for the life-giving miracle of maternal love and I would not deprive myself of gaining a personal experience of the highest happiness that human existence can provide. For the first time in my life I started to look around to find someone to have children with.

I had not been brainwashed by Hollywood stories about romantic fantasies, nor did I care about social status. In my opinion, a responsible man and woman get together to raise a family, not only to have sex or to spend time in social gatherings. Other people dedicate their lives to sex and practice prostitution in different ways, married or not. They feel forced to act and focus their interest in the lowest instincts.

In my opinion, a fulfilling relationship involves having children and educating them. This great responsibility lasts twenty or more years and does not consist only in having fun in bed. When I decided to have a family, I was not looking for any romantic adventure, nor for money or social advantages, but for a solid, not corrupted, honest partner.

I must have made a list of requirements for such a candidate, somehow in my subconscious. Certainly, he needed to be an outdoor and sport person, he must like adventures, and I must trust him in intelligence, daring, and strength. He must be healthy, not drinking, not smoking and a lover of nature.

Well, as the story goes, when you truly look for something with deep conviction, you will find it. It happened, as I wanted.

Establishing a Family and Professional Success

As soon as I established my self in Caracas, I bought a kayak. I had been hiking and kayaking in Canada, in the large wilderness and lakes north of Toronto; now, I dreamed to paddle in the Caribbean Sea, visiting the beaches along the coast.

One Saturday morning I drove to the coast, downloaded all my equipment on the beach, and started preparing my first short expedition into the sea. I was planning to paddle along the coast to another nearby beach that was not accessible by car, sleep there, and return to my car the next morning. I had a hammock, some water, food, and few other useful items. The weather was wonderful.

Suddenly someone walked on the beach toward me. It was a good-looking young man carrying a full equipment for underwater diving.

He left it nearby and, walking closer, he addressed me saying:

"Where are you going with that kayak?"

"To Playa El Limon" I said.

"It is a nice kayak, he said, where did you got it?"

Well, that is how it all started.

My new friend was an ex-national champion of kayak in his homeland in Europe. He was a healthy looking, friendly person, lover of sports and outdoors.

We quickly got involved in personal experiences of kayaking, underwater diving, hiking, and other sports. We became close friends. No drinking, no smoking, enjoying traveling, sports, and open air.

During the next few months we had an incredible wonderful time kayaking along the beaches on weekends, doing scuba diving (I also bought my equipment) and exploring the northern wild coasts of Venezuela in his jeep.

Shortly after, he got his commercial pilot license and bought a small airplane, a single motor Piper, build with fabric and wood. It was a real antique in aviation, but perfectly functional for our needs and safety.

What a thrill to fly that little light plane! We could go anywhere, land anywhere, and explore every corner. We certainly did fly and explore. We visited every corner in the west and south of Venezuela! He was a wonderful flight navigator and pilot and I fully trusted his skills.

Our friendship became solid and deep. We decided to get married and to start a family. That was a wonderful decision!

I was teaching and working at the University Hospital as specialist in Gynaecology and Obstetrics. I was attending my private clinic and I had a good clientele.

My husband was as a commercial pilot with a private company. He also had his own private business with two employees and two small airplanes for chartering.

We rented a nice house and we bought some land to start building our own home. Adeline came back to Venezuela to live with us in Caracas.

My first baby was born in 1962 and my second one in 1963.

All my dreams had been completely fulfilled!

I had two wonderful healthy babies, and a nice family.

My mother came for a long visit, and also my stepfather visited us.

My profession continued to be very successful, but allowed me to stay sufficient time in the company of my children. I would be at the hospital or at the university in the morning from seven to one. Then, I would come back and play with the children until five in the afternoon. Afterward I would go to my private clinic until nine at night.

My life was well organized and not too stressful, but something suddenly went very wrong.

Second Part:

My Struggle in Caracas

The call of death and
the dark night of the soul
Not all bad things are really bad
It all depends of what we make of them.

Times of war:
The battle against the invasive cancer of the thyroid

The sad surprise

During the Fall of 1964, I started to feel extremely tired. At first I lost weight very fast, became unable to read or concentrate and then I started to gain weight because of water retention. My eyes, hands, and feet were swollen and I had a persistent headache.

Clinical tests showed that I had lost most of my thyroid function. The symptoms were of profound hypothyroidism.

Further test suggested that my thyroid gland was invaded by a malignant tumour that expanded to lymph nodes in the right side of my neck.

The final diagnosis was invasive cancer of the thyroid.

The only treatment was a radical surgery of the neck.

The prognosis was a survival of three months to three years, as the tumour was very advanced and distant bone metastases were suspected.

I was 39 years old.

Fortunately, Adeline had already passed away, serenely during the night, about one year before all this happened.

When the world so suddenly and radically changes around you, it is impossible to realize the magnitude of the disaster until some time later. The first awareness was about my self-image. I was not a healthy person anymore, but a sick person about to die. This was unbelievable.

During all my life I had seen myself as a strong human being. I had been capable of overcoming difficulties and obstacles. I had been skilled in performing professional tasks with responsibility and my body was fit to satisfy my love for sports, outdoor life, and natural challenges. How could I possibly be a sick person? How could I be someone who had been carrying a malignant tumour for a few years without noticing anything? Obviously, the human body has an enormous capacity to adjust. Until a small portion of my thyroid was functional, the metabolic balance was maintained. When the last part of the gland became invaded, the whole biologic system suddenly collapsed.

The mechanism of denial is very powerful in every patient. We tend to suspect that something was wrong in the tests, or that someone made a mistake. For me this period of denial was very short. The clinical evidence was overwhelming. I was not myself anymore. I could feel a great debility setting in and I could imagine what would be like to go through the following step of debilitation and the final crumbling of vitality.

There is no point in trying to "think on something else"; no word of consideration or of support can reach you in these moments. You plunge into an extraneous world in which your previous personality is erased. You loose the memory of what was real before and start struggling to grasp an understanding what is real now.

During the months of October and November 1964, while all the tests were being done, I was feeling extremely tired, but could not imagine the severity of the diagnosis. I continued to work as usual, even if I started to live on coffee and aspirin to support my feebleness.

During the month of December, I took a vacation.

The lab technician at the Central Hospital delivered to me the final results just before Christmas.

"The diagnosis is cancer, and it is invasive!" he said.

I remember the shock and the total absolute silence inside me on becoming aware of the reality of the diagnosis. The world disappeared; I was totally alone in a vast emptiness. Nothing existed, nor did I care. Nothing could reach me.

I drove away from the hospital like in a trance. I parked the car downtown somewhere and started to walk. I was unable to think, unable to function in any rational way. I felt like an automaton, I was walking by putting one foot in front of the other.

The very first awareness that marked my return to a certain degree of consciousness was the intense sunshine and the heat. I realized that it was about two in the afternoon and the temperature was extremely high in those downtown streets of Caracas. I saw myself reflected in the shopping windows like a shadow in the glaring reflexes. I can remember a vivid impression thinking:

"This is how I will be soon, just a wandering shadow in the invisible world!"

The heat forced me to take refuge in a coffeehouse where the air conditioning gave me a pleasant sensation and helped me come back to life. The first conscious thought was:

"I cannot go home and face my children! They will know that something is very wrong; they will know that they lost their mother! I cannot hide my real feelings to them!"

Next, I thought of my husband and decided to call him and ask him to join me where I was. By phone, I mentioned briefly that the condition was very serious. He could not believe it. The poor man came and when I disclosed the diagnosis to him, he was astonished and without words as I was. We were both totally destroyed by the new situation, by the possibility that I would be dead in three months. Then, I asked him to go home and play with the children. I would go for a walk in the park and go home later, when they would be sleeping.

We parted and I drove to the central park.

There was something friendly and reassuring among the huge pines, the grass, and the flowers. The air was fresh and scented, the perfumes of nature started to bring me to life again. I spent several hour wandering around, paying attention to the shapes of trees and flowers, to the fountain, to the little river and the wooden bridge and imagining the attention and dedication of those who designed and cared for the place. My personal problem faded into second place as I was giving attention to the beautiful landscape and to the details of shapes and forms. And then, suddenly, a wave of warm feelings emerged from very deep inside me:

"You don't have to die! The diagnosis is just a medical diagnosis, they tell you the truth, but the outcome depends on you!"

I finally started to cry! What a release of emotions!

"Yes, I said, I will fight! I will fight for my children, for me, for my life! I will fight like a wild beast defends her offspring! I will fight with all my power, with all my art, with all the methods that humans have learned. I will fight in all possible ways!"

I walked and run in that beautiful park, the wave of energy lasted several hours. All my last resources had been mobilized. I felt strong again; I was not going to become a shadow and passively letting go.

"I will call up all the memories of my achievements, all the expressions of who I really am. I will call in my help the love for my children; they will not grow up without the care of a mother! I will never abandon them; they cannot, and will not be the victims of a blind destiny. They are too small to face life alone, they have the right of enjoying the presence of a loving mother!"

My decision became stronger and stronger; the temporary depression had been overcome.

Immediately I started planning the next move in this deadly battle. I needed to get in touch with the wilderness again. We would fly south to the jungle, to the wild territory in the southeast of Venezuela, to the Gran Sabana and the Angel's waterfall. From the power of nature untamed, I will gather the strength for standing the difficult and long surgical procedure, I will obtain the energy for a fast recovery, and I will find my emotional balance again. I will call in my help all the will for survival intrinsic in any living creature. I will change my life stile as needed, I will obey the most useful discipline, I will never give up, this struggle is forever, and I will win!

With this resolve in mind, a few days later, we flow south in our aircraft and we spent several weeks in the wonderful region of the Ayantepuy Mountain, in the southeast of Venezuela.

La Gran Sabana is a vast area that could be reached only by air. At that time, there were neither access roads nor towns. There was only a large Christian Mission of Franciscan Fathers that we had visited on several other occasions, as both my children were baptized there together with several little natives' girls and boys.

For that trip south, we embarked on our private two-motors, Aero-commander. The two children, my mother, my husband, and myself. My mother was visiting us at that time, but I did not tell her anything about my health problem. It was great to have her along in the trip, as she would take care of the children and we had more freedom, my husband, and me, for going on a hike. We stayed at a rural refuge-hotel in a place called Canaima, run by a Dutch friend of us called Rudy and his wife. They had two little girls and the four children were happy playing together under the supervision of my mother.

The Ayan-tepuy is a spectacular mountain rising alone about 6,000 feet from the plains between two huge rivers. All around is the tropical jungle. Strange as it may be, there is an abundant source of water emerging on top of this isolated mountain from the depth of the earth. The water runs among deep canyons on the summit of the mountain until it reaches the vertical cut edge of the rocks. From there, the water falls freely for one kilometre down to the forest. It is a spectacular waterfall and it is the highest in the world. It was discovered at the beginning of last century by an American bush pilot called Angel. The name of the waterfall is now Angel's Fall.

Our friend Rudy was the only one at that time who dared to organize expeditions reaching by river the foot of the waterfall. It involved crossing rapids and doing portages in the most difficult conditions, but it was an exhilarating adventure. We had done it before and on this trip, we were only looking for a peaceful environment. My husband and myself, we hiked on trails that Rudy had opened in different directions from his hotel. The magic of the tropical forest was present in all its power and I felt most energized by it.

During the evenings, we enjoyed the good meals and the company of children and adults. It was a perfect match of solitude and company. I forgot everything unpleasant and felt great joy to be surrounded by the full power of nature and by the greater emotional links that I had in my life, my children, my husband and my mother. It was a perfect time!

The father of Rudy was also present at the hotel, visiting his family for a few weeks. He lived in Amsterdam and was a retired university professor of physics, an interesting person. We ended up with deep discussions on physics, philosophy, and the new age.

We were sitting there, deep into the tropical jungle and far remote from all the so called civilized life, but we could not ignore the ferment and the new paths that started to open up for human evolution. It was the end of 1964, the time of the hippie's revolution in the USA, the time of the Beatles revolution in pop music, the time of students' unrest everywhere in the world, the time when most people tried to understand the concepts behind Einstein's relativity, the time when we all thought that a new world was emerging.

However, my concrete reality of the moment was to get ready for a big surgery!

The radical operation of the right neck

I came back to Caracas ready for the operation.

The surgical procedure lasted 6 hours.

When I opened my eyes, I felt that I was dying.

I was in bed, in a private room at the hospital. My bed was facing a window and I could see the bright blues sky of Caracas in a sunny morning. I was barely conscious and could not move, as I was surrounded by cushions supporting my arms and my head. The intravenous drip was slowly entering my system keeping away the pain and the full awareness. In the complete silence of the room, I could hear my breath, shallow and fast, coming out noisily through the tracheotomy. I tried to swallow and it was very painful. I did not try again. I could see my hands, stretched at both sides of my body, but I could not see my arms. Moving my head was impossible.

A nurse entered the room quickly, took my pulse, controlled the dripping, looked at my face, did not say anything, and left.

I closed my eyes, the only thing that I could move, and tried to make sense of the whole story.

A little voice inside me suggested:

"Why did you accept to do this surgery, when you know that you must die anyhow?"

I became more clearly aware of my little complaining ego and asked:

"What did you say?"

"You know what I said," the little voice repeated, "what is the point of doing this surgery? Don't you feel how much it hurts? It is easier just to be dead."

At this point, I woke up:

"NO! You are wrong! NO, I am not going to die! I am not going to abandon my children just like this, letting go and die! You are wrong! I will never give up! I will fight, I will be strong! I will be stronger than the cancer cells! I will kill them all they are not going to kill me! Now the surgery has taken away all my neck on the right side where the cancer was more invasive; only a few malignant cells are left in my body, I will not allow them to survive and kill me. This is a life or death battle and I will win! Stop complaining and whining!"

I got excited and my breath became noisy and fast until I choked.

I tried to cough, but it was impossible, I was suffocating.

Some alarm must have gone on because a nurse rushed in, she pushed a tube with aspiration inside the tracheotomy and finally some air reached my lungs. Life came back with oxygen in my blood.

I learned a lesson. For the moment, be quiet. Leave the fighting for later. I closed my eyes again, paid attention to my rhythmic breathing and relaxed as much as I could.

I remembered the last days before the operation. We went to the Amazon, to hike in the jungle, to absorb the strength of Nature untamed. My husband and me, we went on long walks along the Caroni River on small hiking paths that our friend Rudy had prepared for his guests. The sceneries were majestic and the temperature pleasant under the thick cover of the high vegetation along the river.

We were alone in the depth of the forest and we shared the precious moments of beauty and peace. We both were aware of the seriousness of the situation. The diagnosis of invasive cancer of the thyroid left no doubts. Malignant cells invaded all the lymph nodes on the right side of my neck and shoulder. According to the experience of the surgeons and clinicians, the cancer would soon invade the bones, mostly of the spine, or other organs and then quickly spread all over the system. The prognosis was very bad. The cancer would kill me in a few months, if I did not want a radical surgery.

If I accepted a very broad radical surgery, removing as much as possible of damaged tissues such as muscles of the neck and shoulder, lymphatic, vessels, nerves and all fat tissues, the probabilities of surviving could increase up to two or three years. But, at what cost of pain and distress! Nothing else could be done. No other treatments could be effective.

We talked very deeply, in profound communion among our selves and with nature. Human sympathetic interaction is one of the greatest gifts of being able to talk, expressing feelings and thoughts and understanding each other in depth. I received great support from my husband and he was able to reinforce my decision and my own courage.

It had been a relaxing, pleasant vacation and I had gathered a lot of strength for the difficult decision that I had to take in January about the radical surgery. Some preliminary Lab tests were done. I took a prolonged leave from work at the university. I named a substitute for my medical duties. All was done automatically without telling anybody why.

Then, days had gone-by fast, and now here I was, trying to survive the damages of the knife and of the blood loss. Why should all this happen? What is the meaning of this intense suffering? What is the meaning of life? The whole thing does not make sense. I have accomplished all my duties, I studied, graduated, specialized and finally now I have a wonderful family.

I have not harmed anybody, why must I be punished like this?

My little whining ego jumped up again:

"You see, I told you not to accept the surgery!"

"Shut up you little ignorant, selfish and fearful, let me think deeper, I want to understand what is going on, I want to know, I want to be clear, no matter what happens, but I need to make sense of all this!"

The door opened and the head nurse came in. She was a good friend of mine and we had shared many difficult cases in the operating room. I tried to smile. She had a gentle deep look.

"Doctor Francini, you are coming along fine. You are now in intensive care and cannot receive any visitor, but your husband and some friends are waiting for you to recover more and visit you.

You cannot talk because you have a tracheotomy and a tube in your trachea, so I brought you some paper and a pencil if you want to tell us something, you can write a note.

Your surgeon will come to visit you as soon as the lab report about the histology of the lymph nodes is delivered to him."

She paused then she added:

"All the nurses think on you and we are all at you bed side!"

Emotion overcame me and I wanted to cry, but I could not, I was too weak even for that. She pressed my hand in sympathy, increased the intravenous dripping, and left. I plunged in deep sleep.

When I opened my eyes again, the early dawn was painting the sky with some grey and some pinkish. The dripping was running slow and all my body was aching, but my brain was alert because I had heard a voice. Some soft, gentle words resonate in my head: "Perdónate, perdona, y aprende a amar." ("Forgive your self, forgive, and learn to love.")

I repeated these words and asked: "Who talked?" Maybe it was the nurse who came in the room to change the intravenous dripping. But, it was unlikely. "Forgive and learn to love." No, it was more precise, it said: "Forgive yourself." "Yes, I know what this means! I can remember clearly the scenery!"

My memory raced back many, many years. It was war time in Rome, we had no water and that day I was lucky to find a distribution tank. I had been on line for hours with my bucket. Now it was full and I was walking toward home very carefully, not to spill it. Suddenly, a young wounded Nazi soldier was in front of me. He was injured on the head and face and the dried blood was covering his neck and chest. It was a terrible sight of extreme suffering and horror. He must have run away from the battlefield just south of my house in Rome. He was a fugitive and the military police would shot him anywhere they would find him. He was a boy of my age, a teenager. His eyes were fixed on the water in my bucket. He was thirsty and dying of his infected wounds. I gathered some water in my hands and he drank with feverish anxiety, more and more water, then turned around and slowly walked away to hide and die in some building ruined by the bombing.

In that moment, I hated God! How could he permit so much suffering! Where was that benevolent Being that I used to know when I was a child? Why so much cruelty? Why that carnage of young lives in the battle of Montecassino? Why the destruction of a whole continent and fifty two million dead?

Yes, I remembered, I hated God, I judged the suffering of humanity on my own standard. I went home to cry and despair. My old faith was gone. From that day on, for more than twenty years, I had never forgotten the cruelty, the horrors of the war. The Nazi occupation, the killing, the bombing.

Now, I was in pain and almost dying. Now, I had to forgive!

I had to forgive myself for hating God. I had to forgive others for creating the hell of the war with their personal egoism, selfishness, and greed.

I must forgive, forgive! I must forgive the torturers, the most evil ones. Forgive the gas chambers, the holocaust, the hatred, and the fear!

Not only I had to forgive, I must learn to love.

Not only love my family, but just love, love humanity, the entire world, without judgements, without attachments. What a task!

I forgot myself and my pain in the vision of the past and in the understanding of the whole world struggle.

That insight lasted a long time. I was not thinking. No reasoning could help me in any way. I was confronting a reality too big for me to cope. In the mist of my stupor and confusion, it was clear that my recovery was related to my inner transformation.

I knew that it was necessary to develop an unending desire for growth and development; that I had to change the rusty aspects of my inner self as much as I could; but, this new insight requiring a cosmic forgiveness from the depth of my heart, was something incredibly vast and demanding! The cancer and the radical operation were not a punishment, but a need for purification of the resentment that I had let grow in my heart.

It was my unavoidable reality!

"I must forgive myself for allowing hatred to enter my heart. Not only because I hated God itself, but because I hated the whole universe and everybody in it! I separated myself from my racial karma. I run away from Italy to Venezuela, to get away from the problem of my resentment. I carried that profound emotional wound for twenty years trying to delete it from my memory, but it was there all the time!

Now, if I want to recover, the only path open to me is total, profound forgiveness. I cannot judge the universal Laws.

From a physical point of view, I am not free. Only at a spiritual level I am totally free. Only by purifying my negative thoughts can I reach a higher spiritual plane!"

I was dealing with these profound issues, when the little voice of my ego started again:

"You are so philosophical and you don't understand that after all this you will become just a corpse anyhow. No matter how much effort you build in for escaping your terrestrial destiny, still, you are just a corpse! I know how much work you are giving me with this surgery! I know it, because am ruling all your subconscious system! All is for nothing because you will become a corpse anyhow! You could have spared me this useless work!"

I reacted strongly:

"Be sure that I don't listen to you at all! I ignore you completely!

Do your duty and don't complain! After all, if some day we will be able to enjoy the beach and he sun again, it will be because I was brave! It is your duty to support me, your higher Self! Anyhow, it is you who will some day become a corpse, not me! So, be happy to work a little longer!"

I must confess that the idea of becoming a corpse really hit me. The little devilish ego was always able to upset me!

I tried to move and, surprisingly, I could move a bit better. My feet, my legs responded well. I could breath deeply even if the tube in my trachea made a funny noise. I stretched my back slightly an was able to smile:

"Hey, little devil, you are doing your work nicely! I am feeling part of the body again!"

"Thank you "Superior Self!" At your very orders!" said ironically the little voice.

The door opened and the head nurse came in:

"How are you feeling today, Dr. Francini? You look much better and I think that we are going to take you out of intensive care, so you can receive visitors! Do you like that?"

"Yes" I answered by closing my eyes. I certainly could not move my neck or speak!

My husband came and we both cried silently holding hands.

Then, other friends came and finally the surgeon with the histological report. The tumour was a mixed tumour and all the lymph nodes were invaded. Nothing new.

During the next days they kept me busy with rehabilitation and some physiotherapy. I learned how to remove my tracheal tube, clean it, and replace it. I received very pleasant sponge baths. Finally, I got out of bed and was able to look at myself in the bathroom mirror. I looked horrible! The right half of my head had been in part shaved for the operation and my hair were long on the left side. It was impossible to face my children in such conditions!

Fortunately, a young assistant nurse agreed to go with me to a nearby beauty parlour to fix my hair cut, as soon as I was able to walk. I was very worried about how I looked, as I hoped that my children did not found Mom very ugly. I could buy a hat, but I could not wear a hat inside the house, so I hoped for the best. We had told the children that I was attending a medical congress in some nearby country.

When I fully recovered my breathing capacity, a short surgery was needed to close the tracheotomy.

Finally, the day arrived that I could go home! The beauty parlour did a good job and my face looked more or less normal.

That Monday morning my husband picked me up ad we bought some toys before going home. All went well. The only comment that my children made was: "Mommy, you cut your hairs very short!" and then we played with the new toys as we normally did. Life was coming back as usual!

I recovered quickly. Some more tests were done. Radioactive thyroid hormone was used for a full body scanning, but no active metastases were found. That was a good beginning.

I started the treatment with a daily dose of thyroid to balance my metabolism. As all the thyroid tissue was invaded and had been removed, I would be on replacement therapy with a doses of 100 micrograms daily.

Coping with the help of Yoga and Macrobiotic diet

As soon as I recovered, I went back to work as usual at the university, hospital, and private clinic, but I changed my diet and did several other reforms in my life stile. I studied Macrobiotics. I decided to strictly adhere to that method and for the next eighteen years, I followed the Macrobiotic diet and life style.

The memory of the practice of breathing and Yoga exercises that I had done when I was very young came back to me. I remembered the teachings of Yogi Ramacharaca, the little printed books that I found in my parents' bookshelf. I did not have them with me any more, but I remembered the details of the breathing technique and mostly, I remembered the great trust that I had put in those teachings and practices. They helped me healing my kidney infection at that time. I firmly decided that I would resume my daily breathing exercises, very early in the morning, at sunrise, on my balcony. And so I did for many years to follow!

I also started to practice Hata-Yoga regularly together with meditation and visualization. This last exercise consisted in concentrating mentally on visualizing the cancer cells that could have spread into my body. I would bring each cell clearly into my mind's eye, define its characteristics, and then see it losing its shape, shrinking, and die. This was a very rewarding practice, as it gave me the feeling that I was doing something useful by killing the offensive invaders.

The other very pleasant exercises were the breathing practices performed before doing Yoga. It felt very good to breathe deeply, consciously and slowly early in the morning, imagining that all the wastes were released through this purification breathing.

After a certain time it was clear that I had organized my working and daily activities the best that I could from a physical point of view. Next the mental doubts, fears, and anxieties had to be taken care of.

My first reaction to the invasive cancer had been a physical, primitive one, based on the natural instinct of survival. I had mobilized the resources of my animal nature, of the biological being born to survive in the wild. I had felt like a natural product of the most primitive life on earth, gathering all the strength accumulated by ages of survival struggle. This approach had the advantage of producing immediate results, clear and tangible.

I firmly knew that I wanted to live. But, humans have a brain that is not fully satisfied only by material considerations. I needed a philosophical and mental, superior, deeper understanding of the process, in order that my healing would become global. As usual during time of great stress, our emotions go back and forth. Some days we believe that we made it through and the next day we sink back again in despair.

The philosophical battle and the "The dark night of the Soul"

The shock of the diagnosis and the following physical damage produced by the operation to my self-image and self-esteem had been extremely serious. Everything was so unexpected and had happened so fast that I had no time to adjust. Intellectually, I could understand that being angry at my cancer, or recriminating against destiny, or feeling some sort of guilt, were not solutions to my answer:

"Why did this happen?"

Nevertheless, my emotions were stronger than my reason. I felt hatred for the disease, I was happy to mentally kill my cancer cell every day and, mostly, I felt that:

"The whole universe is against me!"

I was left alone, abandoned, struggling in a vast stormy sea!

Hardly being able to keep my head out of water.

I also had a vision of myself hiding inside a huge fortified castle while an army of enemies was trying to reach and kill me. In short, for some times I was at the bottom of a big depression. But, surrender was not in my nature, so I soon became emotionally more aggressive.

I became actively furious against everything. I was eager to find some sort of revenge, against life, against the world. So, I bought an expensive accident insurance for myself in the name of my children. I decided that if metastasis appeared in some region of my body, rather then dying in pain, suffering in a hospital bed, I would create for myself a deadly car accident and at least my children would be rich! I indulged in this idea for months and it helped me a lot. It was a revenge! It was my dear secret and gave me a new strength.

I imagined that I still had a weapon and that I was in control of something, even if not of my life. There are personalities who accept being deprived of everything, if dominated, they submit. On the contrary, the training that life had given me was to fight to the very end. The image that I had of my self was of dying on the battlefield holding a sword in my hand! I shell be dying fighting for what I want; I may give up my life, but not my will!

As soon as I reached this understanding, a deep, old wound opened up inside me. I realized that deep inside me I never forgave my mother for sinking into a deep depression just when her courage was most needed, during the difficult years of the war. Being depressed and remaining in her bed, waiting to be killed by a bomb was the entire example that she had given me. Now, I hated to hide myself in the escape of depression. But, this insight was a new one. I had completely repressed any feelings and judgment about my mother's behaviour. At that time, I had felt that it was her right to be depressed, if that was her choice; I tended to be tolerant and supportive. The reality was that I had felt abandoned in those difficult moments and only the presence of Adeline had given me strength.

That's how I started a long process of analyzing my past. I wanted to bring up to consciousness all the repressed wounds of war, of hatred, of resentment, all that I had pushed down in the depth of the subconscious. I wanted to clean up the emotional landscape once and forever, to the very bottom on the most painful injury.

The self-analysis and the recall of the neck irradiation

Instead of going to an analyst, I used the technique of meditation during one hour in my office every evening after work. I would relax, concentrate and bring to memory my early years, searching for meaningful events. I learned to look at my own past with the eye of a professional. It was an impersonal scientific research. I needed to clear any repressed emotions, any event that had wounded my sensibility and that I had apparently forgotten. I started to write comments on my findings and to dwell as deep as I could with the greatest sincerity.

Soon I found that the sense of being abandoned and rejected had started way back in my early years when I overheard some one saying that I should have been born a boy because my father wanted a boy, but unfortunately I was born a girl and it had been a great deception for my parents. When I heard these comments, I felt that something must be very wrong with me. I was very young and could not understand the difference between a boy and a girl. It is amazing how inconsiderate adults can be when they believe that young children don't understand. What a great harm their words can produce. Even if at the moment I heard it I could not understand it fully, nevertheless, that imprint of not being wanted was very powerful in later years. Somehow, I concluded that I did not belong to my parents, or to any other social group. Later on, when I was told the story of how Adeline had saved my life when I was born, it confirmed my feelings of not belonging to my parents.

Sitting in my office, during several days I analyzed my discovery and its consequences. It was unbelievable that I could clearly remember such a comment after more than thirty years. Obviously, the finding that I was not wanted had to do with my sense of rebellion that manifested in later years. It also had to do with my being so eager to leave Italy after the war. Getting away from my past meant finding a new freedom. Getting rid of the duty of being with my mother was a liberating experience. The evidence that I was not wanted had never been contradicted during my years in Rome. It was only natural that I wanted to put an end to that unpleasant situation. Philosophers or psychologists may say that I left my hometown under a 'compulsion' and therefore it was not an act of free will. This would be wrong. I managed the situation during more than twenty years. I waited until my mother was married and all was in order. Then, I had the right to choose my new life with an act of free will.

At the time I left, I could only see the horrors of war around me and I attributed to them my desire to leave. Now, my analysis showed to me that my motivation was also deeply moved by my personal condition. I endured for years that rejection until the times were ripe for my liberation. Could that repression have contributed to the development of my cancer? Nobody can know for sure.

Having achieved this insight gave me confidence that deeper analysis would bear positive fruits for the understanding of myself and for the release of any further block in my past.

Further memories of later years brought a surprising vision. I was lying on a small hard bed in a dark room and a frightening large device was looming on top of me and descending toward my face and neck. I was deadly scared, but could not move because I was tight up to the bed. It was a horrible feeling of distress and panic. Why do adult abuse children like that? Suddenly, I knew what it was. I recognized an x-ray device. I had been irradiated on my neck! When did this happen? I wrote an urgent letter to my mother asking her at what age I was irradiated and to give me the details. Her letter gave me lots of details. I was nine and a half years old and I had chronic infected tonsils. Some doctor suggested that tonsils could be irradiated and they would shrink making the operation unnecessary. So, several doses of x-ray were given to my neck.

Obviously, that treatment was the origin of my cancer! During the years of 1933-34, doctor still ignored the permanent damages produced by x-ray. Radiation had been used everywhere in Europe to treat chronic infected tonsils. I rushed to consult Medical Journals looking for research on cancer of the thyroid following neck irradiation. There were several articles reporting cancer of the thyroid and of the thymus after irradiation of the tonsils in children. I had found a powerful answer! My cancer was a yatrogenic one! It was the consequence of medical treatment. I was a victim of my own profession.

After this discovery, I discussed the topic with colleagues and they were even more worried than before about the outcome of my condition. The example of the victims of Hiroshima showed that many irradiated children had not survived long. So, I was left on my own to continue my war on cancer.

Getting rid of more conditioning

My evenings' self analysis continued and one day I was hit by the awareness of being too much a slave of being 'the-doctor'. The seven years of specialization and academic training had reinforced that professional aspect of myself, inhibiting all other aspects. I realized that the eco of the paging in the hospitals: "Doctor, an urgent call ..." was constantly present to my subconscious. I had become only 'Doctor' for most of my day. Only from one to five p.m. I was 'Mammy' or was called by my name. The doctor personality was overwhelming. I had to get rid of that.

I remembered how important outdoors life was to my well-being, how much I needed the sunshine, the wind, the shimmering of the sky and the sense of adventure. The duties of the profession and two pregnancies had reduced my participation to sports and physical activity during the last few years. Something had to be done that I could share with the children and with my husband when he was free from his duties as a commercial pilot.

I searched for a house at the beach and I bought one. I got a sailing boat and later a small motor boat for water skiing. My personality started to become more balanced by taking short vacation to the beach, swimming, sailing and relaxing in the sun. And mostly, in the early morning doing my profound breathing and Yoga exercises at the seashore! That was healing and invigorating!

This was only the beginning of my des-personalization. It was a first step, but I needed to go deeply to find my real essence. Now, I could easily handle the -doctor- and the -adventurer-, I could recognize them and bring them to life when I wanted. But, I suspected that many more personalities were hidden in myself.

Some time later, I had another sudden memory. I saw myself hidden under my bed reading "forbidden" books while all my dolls lied abandoned on the floor of my room. This remembrance made me laugh and made me feel happy and safe. I must have been nine or ten years old and I had started stealing books from my parent's library and reading them when nobody was around. I did not like to play with dolls. I found them boring and useless, but I kept receiving presents of dolls. So, I started using them as an excuse to be alone and read. Adeline was in the kitchen, thinking that I was safe in my room playing with dolls, my parents were out somewhere and it was a perfect time for me to read "adults" books. Victor Hugo, Tolstoy, and Dostoievsky were my preferred ones. My parents were giving me children book to read. But, how could I be interested in witches and ogres when I was participating in the human dramas of Anna Karenina, the brothers Karamazoff, the hunchback of Notre Dame, Cosette, and Jean Valjean? At night, I would discuss directly with Tolstoy, or with Victor Hugo their motivations, choices and presentation.

This memory helped me discover in myself the early personality of a literary critic that had been completely submerged by the 'doctor' personality. What a pity! After having that insight I understood that reading, understanding and developing a taste for literature and philosophy was another need, another of my personalities that claimed to be allowed to live and prosper. I promised myself that I would soon do something about that!

There was another aspect of this same behaviour that was not so innocent. I was cheating, I was lying, I was simulating. I had a double game going on. That was something to examine more closely, the 'pretending' to be a good child. Why did I resort to that stratagem? Obviously, I was too much alone and reading was my evasion, my defence, and my search for communication. The society in which I grew up was extremely repressive. Fascism was oppressing everybody and fear was everywhere.

I had no extended family, no friends. All I had was school, homework, dolls, and children books. In the morning, Adeline would help me dress up and gave me breakfast. At night, my mother would help me with some home work and kiss me good night. Very seldom would I go out with my parents. Anyhow, I did not like it because it was extremely boring. For them, the idea of having fun was to go to an expensive restaurant all dressed up, sitting frozen in the chair, have an ice cream or some other fancy mixture supposed to be very fine, shut up, behave, and go home again. I was not considered a human being, but a thing to be educated, like a little dog or monkey. I was not supposed to talk, ask questions or anything at all. In comparison with all this, how wonderful and rich was the life described in my beloved books! How warm and friendly were the heroes and the victims, how trustful the authors! How interesting their conversations, their dramas, their psychology!

Continuing the analysis of my childhood memories, I remembered that beside these books, there were others that fascinated me. They were the books on Yoga, by Yogi Ramacharaka, that I discovered at the bottom of a large bookcase in my parent's studio. I read the one titled "Mystic Christianity" when I was about nine years old and a new dimension of understanding opened up in my life. The message of Jesus was explained in simple easy words and was much more appealing than any other presentation I ever read before. I remember that for weeks I was taken by this book and that I read it many, many times trying to understand it better and deeper.

After my analysis, this memory was so intense that I decide to search in Caracas for that book and read it again. I was lucky and I found it in a new edition. By reading it again, I experienced the same joy as when I was a child. Another book of the same author that I had read as a child was: Lectures on Yoga Philosophy. From that book I had learned about the importance of Prana, the vital energy that permeates everything. I had learned to eat an apple feeling that I was eating the energy of the sun and the strength of the earth. I had learned to perceive food as the result of the effects of light and water, of the fertility of the soil and the shining of the sun. It was a profound experience that I had forgotten, brain washed by years of medical training!.

My years of academic training had almost deleted the concepts of natural life. If I had not dedicated so many evening hours to meditation and to remembering important events of my childhood, I would have remained as I had become, a frozen doctor pasted in medical books.

This idea made me understand that whatever the outcome of my cancer, it had been welcome for allowing me to remember so many interesting things of my past. Now, at forty, I was growing and understanding myself much better.

This is another indication that we cannot consider something, not even a cancer, as completely a bad experience. We cannot know what will be the result of a new situation that forces us to look more closely inside our own self. I also understood that what had been a terrible repression and solitude during my childhood, had been at the same time the opportunity for great discoveries that would not have taken place if I was a child playing happily with other children in a free environment. I had been forced to grow much faster and deeper. This same attitude was an advantage during the years of war when loneliness and physical hardships did no affect me so much as compared with the depression that they caused to others.

I discovered also that I had become able to lie and to manipulate situations very soon in life. I did not condemn others for forcing me to lie. I just thought that it was the way they wanted it. I could not be bored and submit to a life style that was not pleasant for me. My survival strength taught me how to evade the repression in the most peaceful way, silently and privately. Probably from that attitude derived my deep introversion.

Still now, I love to be alone doing interesting activities such as reading, writing, drawing, pottery, or doing gymnastics or listening to classic music. Somehow, I am the same one person as when I was a child, but I have gained a different scope in awareness. When I was younger I would just react to situations, now, at forty, I was able to understand circumstances and consider different approaches and possible solutions.

More meditation and recovery

Day after day at my office, I continued my evening meditations and self-analysis, remembering events from my very early years, to my teenage times. I knew that I could not get out of my own skin. I knew that each one of us is inevitably alone and that it was my duty to re-establish the balance of my body.

I was the one ruling my physiology, my thoughts, and my own moods. The sudden collapsing of my thyroid function had dragged my metabolism and all my systems out of balance. It was my task to re-build the core of my personal structure. I needed to spread the information about myself to every cell, to every department of my physical entity. The cancer had given to my body an impulse toward dissolution and I had to stop sliding toward entropy and death. I had to centre my will and the consciousness of my existence. The will to live had to emanate from the very core of myself as a clear message of order, joy, and awareness.

The experience of a certain degree of emotional self-sufficiency during my early years was very useful when my father got severely sick and later died when I was eleven years old. During the last two years of my father's life, it was very rare for me to be with my parents. They were in and out of hospitals and clinics and when they were at home I was asked to stay in my room and don't make noise. I did not resent my increased solitude, as I went deeper in the study of many writings. By then, I was not hiding any more under my bed to read, as nobody would worry about what I was doing.

My self-analysis during evening hours in my office went on regularly during a few years. Beside the fact that I had been irradiated at the neck, I did not find any other important event that could have contributed to the development of my thyroid cancer. Certainly, irradiation was a sufficient factor.

Every few months I continued to be in control for metastasis, but after five years none was apparent and I was feeling well.

As years passed quickly, my children had grown up, and we enjoyed the house at the beach, swimming, motor boat, sailing boat, and water skiing with lots of friends of their age.

Work and family life were pleasant and fulfilling.

Nevertheless, my old post-traumatic stress disorder had not improved. I still sometimes remembered the war and its horrors. The old question that I used to address to that benevolent being, was always the same: "Why did you allow so much suffering, so much destruction, so much hatred?" "How is it possible that Goodness and Beauty were deleted from the face of the Earth for five long years of hell?" The image of young soldiers wounded and hopeless, wandering in the streets to die in any corner, kept coming back again, and again. I needed to recover a faith that the war had taken away from me.

Third Part:

The Spiritual Quest

I am grateful to the supreme wisdom
Of ancient India, the land of spiritual
Masters, of Gandhi and of Yoga!

Times of peace
Searching for answers: "Who am I?"
"Why the horrors of the war?"

Study and meditation

Beside the work and family life, it was extremely important for me to dedicate attention to my spiritual development. The shock of the invasive cancer and the close touch with death forced me to ask "Who am I?" "What am I?" "Am I just a corpse?" "Is there a spiritual dimension?"

"If there is a spiritual dimension, if there is something subtler than gross materialism, then, how can the horrors of war be explained?"

These questions were the beginning of a serious spiritual quest.

For many years I dedicated the little free time I had to study spiritual texts. It was very relaxing to break the stress of the day by reading at night, when the children were peacefully sleeping in their rooms.

During many years, I seriously dedicated my attention to Western Mysticism; I took a correspondence course with B.O.T.A. and followed the teachings of Paul Foster Case in Alchemy and Cabbala. I studied the writings of Dionne Fortune and others inspired authors. I also enjoyed the wonderful books by Yogananda Paramhansa, as well as deepening all aspects of Yoga: Raja, Gnana, and Bakti, in the writing of Swami Vivekananda.

I meditated regularly; went deep into meditation of my own death, continued to perform breathing exercises, Hata-Yoga and followed strictly my macrobiotic diet. At the same time I also studied other Eastern teachings such as, Buddhism by Suzuki, Taoism in the translations of Clearly, the Tao of Laotze, the I Ching by Wilhelm, and other inspired texts. I also participated in group studies and workshops.

I realized that the basic understanding of spiritual evolution in all continents, times, and cultures are fundamentally the same. Nevertheless, I felt that something was missing. I could understand all the teachings intellectually, but I, myself, was not truly transformed. After more then ten years following the neck operation, I was still searching for that complete realization that I knew was eluding me. Then, it suddenly happened.

One patient of mine, phoned me to invite me to her house for a session of changing and meditation. She told me that she had found a great Yoga teacher and she was sure that I would like the chanting, the music, and the tapes. On the day of the meeting, I went to her house. As I was the first guest to arrive, she asked me to wait in the sitting room while she prepared some refreshments in the kitchen.

The sitting room had a warm, intimate feeling, with cushions on the floor, candles, flowers, and burning incense. I sat down and made myself comfortable. Immediately I felt a wave of happiness and I looked around.

In front of me, hanging on the wall was a picture showing the face of a middle-aged man. I imagined that it was the photograph of the Master of Yoga, so I got up to look at it more closely.

> *I looked in his eyes and he looked at me. I went blank.*
> *I knew him! He was my own self! His picture was the picture of me!*
> *I stared at him loosing the sense of time, of location and of everything.*
> *He smiled at me. I answered: "Who are you? Why do I know you?"*
> *Then, suddenly I knew! "You have overcome the fear of death!"*
> *He smiled again at me with intelligent eyes.*
> *Recognition was complete; a link for-ever had been established.*

When other guests arrived, we had the chanting session and I was flying. Something, way beyond my understanding, was going on inside me.

I borrowed some books by the Teacher from my friend and went home to read about his message. I read and meditated all night. In the morning, I pretended to be sick and excused my self from work for the whole day. I needed rest and solitude.

The message of Swami Muktananda Paramahamsa for me was very simple:

"*God dwells in you as you*"

His words hit me with incredible power.

"*See God in each other*"

This was his suggestion for all social interactions.

That was all. He would quote scriptures, poets, ancient saints, stories and words of songs to comment on these two teachings. But, that was it.

"When you fully absorb the fact that you have been willed by God, that He actually 'dwells in you as you', then, no matter what happens to you, all is natural, and you are at rest, just peace!
Once you fully incorporate this teaching, then, you know that other humans also have been willed by God, so you just see God in them, no matter what they do or say.
No need to struggle, no need to judge, just remember God with all your love at every breath, at every heart-beat.
Drop the thorns, breath calmly and be grateful!"

"You manifest your inner God, as you!"
"But, you must be aware and awake!" would comment Swami Muktananda in his writings!

That was it. Light out of the tunnel. I must se him! I must talk to him! I must absorb his teachings directly from him!

For the first time in my life, I had a glimpse of *'Unconditional Love'! Of true God's Love! Of that universal and intimate Love, that deeply nurtures our Soul!*

Traveling to India and meeting Gurudev Swami Muktananda

Some time later, a sudden trip to India landed me in Bombay. I had discovered that there was an international conference in Bombay on 'Interpersonal Psychology'. The main speakers were well known western psychologists, philosophers, Mother Theresa and Shree Swami Muktananda Paramahamsa.

Thousand of people from all over the world were attending.

I was one of them, but, as I just arrived from Caracas, I was very confused by the crowd and by the new Indian environment.

I saw Mother Theresa and listen to her wonderful holy words.

Next, Swami Muktananda delivered a profound speech linking East/West traditions and highlighting his "Meditation Revolution" for the development of a broader intercontinental understanding and personal growth. His words increased my desire and determination to get to know him closer. I had no idea about how this could happen.

Then, I read a big poster that said:

"Swami Muktananda invites all participants to the Congress to visit his Ashram on occasion of the Shivaratri Sapta celebrations. The busses are offered by the Ashram and will depart at the end of the Congress."

The next week I was in Ganeshpuri, at the Ashram. It was the annual celebration of Shivaratri, the Festival of Lights. There were four thousand people at the Ashram the day I arrived there. The air was saturated with melodious chanting, incense, and perfumes.

That day I felt the presence of the spiritual Master in the form of the entire landscape, of the many elegant buildings and of the park and the trees. He created all this, where there was only a sun-dried desert. All the buildings and the gardens were first in his mind. What a work of art! I lost completely myself in it.

I remember that I sat down and listen to the melodious chanting and to the drumming for a long time. I could not join the chanting, in those first days, as my voice would not come out. During the rest of the week I enjoyed walking slowly across the gardens, still listening to the music that was softly echoing everywhere. There were great peace, joy, and love all around me.

A week later Gurudev was giving 'darshan', resting in a beautiful patio and talking to visitors. He was sitting under the trees across the temple, surrounded by shining white marbles, teaching, answering to people, smiling and blessing everyone. I can still see him very clearly in my memory, from where I was standing in the corridor close to the offices.

I had a little gift for Baba Muktananda. It had been hanging on my neck during the trip from Venezuela, but I did not dare to go close to him. It took me another week before I was able to take the decision and line up for the 'darshan'. That was the monumental event that transformed forever my life.

The fundamental question that I had in mind was:
"What am I?"
The quest for this answer had been the leading interest during my long years of study. As a scientist submitted to a materialistic cultural environment I had not been able to break the links with my background. According to my Western outlook, the only possible answer to the question was:
"You are a corpse."
Certainly, the influence of the practice and study of Yoga, of the courses on Mysticism, Kabala, Zen, and others, had contributed to broaden my inquiry into the realm of spirituality, but the attachment to the traditional western thinking was still predominant in my mind. I never had any transcendental experience

strong enough to justify a change in the current beliefs related to my profession. Spirituality was a theory and a possibility, but not a reality for me.

When I approached Baba, this query:
"What am I?"
Was in my mind while I was on line waiting for my turn to greet him.

Then, when I finally reached him, I bowed and offered the little gift, saying that all the people in our group in Caracas, Venezuela, asked for his blessings. He said:

"You have undertaken a long journey. You are very welcome and I am happy to see you here! Blessings are extended to all your friends in Caracas, family and relatives!"

Then I asked him to consecrate me, to give me a spiritual name and bestow initiation on me with the sacred ritual of shaktipat. He looked at me in silence, put his hands over my head, touched my forehead, and pronounced some mantras. Then, he searched in a large basket containing several nametags, until he found the name that he wanted for me.

He gave me the tag and looking intensely in my eyes, he asked:
"What is your request?"

I focused in his eyes and suddenly my mind went completely blank, my eyes locked in his. The silence and immobility lasted for some time, I don't know for how long. I can only remember the profound depth of His eyes! He continued with the consecration ceremony, then, he said:

"You have my blessings!"

At that point I was floating in ecstasies. Someone helped me get up and walk away.

I went to my dormitory and slept there for three days.

A bottle of water was put to my bedside and I scarcely had the strength to go to the bathroom. It was a deep, restful sleep without any dream. I suspect that my entire system was rebuilt during those three days.

When I woke up, I felt completely awake and well. The girls in the dormitory looked at me with a little smile:

"You had a good rest!" they said.

"Yes, I said, I don't know what happens, but I could not get up."

They laughed saying that it was the 'Baba effect' and that it also happened sometime to other people.

"Don't worry, they said, you will be fine."

The reality of the fact started to become clear to me. I was not sick, but I had been sleeping for three days with no clinical reason. Certainly, strange for a medical mind!

Next, I got into the routine of the Ashram feeling well and strong and did not think about it any more.

Everyday we would start with one-hour meditation at four a.m. followed by a cup of Chaia tea and chanting for another hour. After breakfast, we would do the work assigned to each and before lunch we would chant again. From one to three in the afternoon we would sleep, as usual in tropical countries, because of the heat of the day. The afternoon work lasted a couple of hours, followed by supper and evening chanting until about ten.

I never had a personal talk or interaction with the Guru again, even if he participated in all the chanting sitting in his chair at the end of the hall. Nevertheless, a new awareness started to dawn in me. The door of communication with the Master Within had been open and I felt the awakening of a new presence.

About a week later, the words of the main Mantra started to repeat it self automatically in my mind while I was busy in the kitchen or in the yard. I noticed this event with some joy thinking that I was really integrating myself into the atmosphere of the Ashram. As I was pleased with this finding, suddenly other words became clear in my mind following each repetition of the Mantra. The new words were: "Eternidad Viviente" ('Living Eternity'). I did not recall hearing these words anywhere before, but the repetition went on automatically in my mind while I was peeling potatoes, or sweeping the patio, together with the Mantra. I could not understand what 'Living Eternity' meant, but they continued to be present in my mind.

The awakening experience at the Ashram

One day I went for a walk in the park of the Ashram. There was a little hill toward the west from where it was possible to enjoy the sunset. There was nobody around and all was beautiful and calm. I decided to take a break in my duties and enjoy the peace of the moment. When I sat there I could not imagine that a total breakthrough in my evolution would shortly occur.

The following is a poetry that I wrote about that day:

> The big statue of Hanuman stands on the hill.
> It was late afternoon and I was resting there.
> Trees, flowers and grass covered

The easy slope down to the valley.
The sun was setting and the air was calm.
I remembered your words, dear Gurudev,
"*There is so much love in the back of your head,*
That you could fill the world with it!
Learn to experience Love! See the Self everywhere!"
With open eyes I lapsed into a state
Of meditation and silence.
The sun went slowly down and
The landscape was shimmering
With soft and warm colours.
A surge of intense happiness and love
Emerged from inside me and spread all around.
Surprised, my mind woke up and asked:
"Where do so much beauty and love come from?"
The Self in me listened to the question
And answered with a gentle smile:
"*This love is radiating into the entire place*
From all of your being.
The Divine is manifesting itself through you.
Under Its spell, all what is visible will grow beyond itself.
It will extend into the invisible
And find its roots into the cosmic order.
'Natural Life' and 'Spiritual Essence'
Are one and the same, but appear separated.
When you bring them together,
With your Love and Intention,
The glory of their blessings spreads over the world."
The sun went down and the colours changed
Into brilliant pink, orange, violet and red.
A symphony of joy, wonder and silence!
"Thank you Hanuman!"

While I was in such an ecstatic mood, suddenly the words 'Living Eternity' became clear to me. It was the answer to my quest:
"What am I?"
"You are 'Living Eternity'" answered Baba to my subconscious query.
"Yes! You are right Baba! Everything that exists is Living Eternity!'"

'Eternity' is out of time and out of space, Eternity is all there is, since ever and for ever. Eternity is all around us, is the only true reality. The Absolute Eternal Truth is from where we all come.

> *"I am Living Eternity, You are Living Eternity, and everything is the manifestation of Living Eternity!"*

An Eternity that is dynamic Consciousness, alive, fully aware, changing, manifesting in the thousand things, creating, maintaining, and renewing the universe!

Eternity that is God and Life and Light and Goodness and Past, Future and Present, all at the same time.

Eternity that is Omniscient, All-Powerful, Infinite and Unique. Eternity that is the whole of all there IS!

How confused I had been, unable to see the evidence of my real being!

The "corpse" is just a dense, biological aspect of the same all pervasive Eternal structure. My human consciousness is just a reflex of the eternal, present, Cosmic Consciousness.

I have a biological body adapted to survive in this terrestrial environment; a body that is the result of million of years of changes and transformations; a body that is the vehicle for the Essence.

This Essence is the Eternal Essence that pervades all Creation.

All this awareness came to me in a flash, with such intensity that I could not cope with all of it and I started to cry and tremble in ecstasy! Suddenly, I could visualize Gurudev, full body, smiling, just in front of me!

"Thank you! Thank you, Baba!

This is the answer I have been waiting for during all my life!"

I remember that the emotion brought about by this new freedom, by this wonderful insight was overwhelming and I could not stop crying. I was crying of joy, of surprise, of gratitude, of liberation, of wonder, of everything and of nothing specific at the same time.

I felt that it was an exceptional moment and not the time to perform my duties. Instead, I went deeper into the park and started to run, to dance, to jump ... I felt that wings were growing on my back and that I could fly, expand, embrace the worlds, the galaxies, the stars, the black holes and the quasars ... I was everything and everything was me!

Some passing swamis smiled saying:

"You got it!"

"Yes, Yes! I got it!"

Now I understood! I profoundly experienced the new universe that opened up. A universe that was there, close by, all the time, but that I was unable to see before. Everything, myself, all my life acquired a new meaning, a deeper sense, and a clear purpose. I had lived in a doubt, an uncertainty, a questioning, a lack of satisfaction, and suddenly, now, all had been answered, all was shining clear, and all was bright and transparent.

I had entered the world of "certainty." I cannot explain what that meant exactly in words, but the full awareness of a new total and global consciousness was a fact for me.

After the first surprise, the firsts hours of crying and discovering a new dimension of existence, I calmed down and went chanting as usual in the evening. The whole aspect of the temple, the voices, the incense, and the decorations were brighter than usual and I enjoyed the ceremony more than ever because it had a clear new meaning.

> *"Yes! I am Living Eternity, All is Living Eternity!*
> *Cosmic Consciousness is the Universal All!"*

When bed-time arrived I was exhausted and fell asleep like a stone, but at dawn I woke up with a terrible nightmare, remembering the war. The horror and the pain were vivid, my emotional wounds were bleeding and torn open again, giving me a painful cramp in the stomach. I covered my head under the blanket and started crying again asking Baba the real stressful, dramatic, question that had constantly poisoned my life for forty years:

"Baba, why the war? Why so much destruction and cruelty?

Why so much suffering? Why all of it?"

After formulating the question and asking for help, I calmed down and fell asleep again. Shortly after I woke up in a jump, I had just had the most incredible dream! A dream that answered for ever the awful questions that had tortured me for years.

I saw myself on a high platform looking down in front of me. At my right side was someone very tall, benevolent, and bending toward me. He was extending his right arm in front and telling me to look at the scene below the platform. I saw people, many, many people walking in circles from the left toward the right. It was like a grey river of people, all close to one another, all walking together, coming from the left side, passing below the platform were I was standing and continuing their march toward the right side. Then, they were turning in a counter-clockwise fashion in a large arch.

As soon as the first people completed the circle, they were suddenly swallowed by a whirlpool that opened up among them in the middle of the circle, completing a spiral movement. The vortex in the centre was deep and black and the new comers were constantly disappearing into it.

I got very upset and screamed to my companion:

"Tell them to stop! They are all going to fall into the vortex! Stop them!"

And I wanted to jump into the crowd to stop their fatal march.

Suddenly, in front of me there was a barrier of high flames.

My companion and myself were separated from the multitude by a big red fire all around us. I looked at him in mute stupor.

He shook his head saying:

"This is how it is."

"That's how it is?" I repeated without understanding.

"Yes, he said, "This is how it is, for those who live only in the body and for the body."

I contemplated the silent march of the crowd. The vortex in the middle of the spiral continued to swallow in its bleakness, waves, and waves of people. The march continued unchanged, monotonous at the same pace, steady, indifferent, inevitable. I was horrified, but I lowered my head because I understood:

"This is how it is!"

At this point, I woke up sweating.

This is how it is in the war!

I remembered. The same sense of inevitable fatality, of total powerlessness, of global indifference, of cold, absolute despair. The same constant movement empty of any meaning, hour after hour, day after day; meaningless life, from an empty past toward a useless future.

The torment of my repressed suffering twisted my body in agony.

In a brief moment the spasm of suppressed anger, misery and anguish became a visible monster that had been threatening to swallow me for ages.

I cried with silent convulsions while the other girls in the dormitory were going to meditation. I remained in bed and could not move.

The transformation of my universe was total and too traumatic to pretend that I could also cope with the daily routine.

This is the outcome of the Guru's Grace. The real Guru is inside each one of us, but we need commitment, concentration, and dedication, to bring the Grace to express itself fully.

The real Guru is inside you! He is The Master Within!

He knows what you need, His benevolence is absolute. His commitment to your welfare is total. He lives for you and continues to be your friend forever, no matter where you are, who you are or what you are. You only need to trust Him completely, totally, from the depth of your heart.

His subtle Divine Energy will support you forever.

The physical Guru is the channel for the Divine Grace that permits us to connect with our inner Self, the Eternal Guru-Principle that is inside each one of us. The awareness of the communication between the Immortal Superior Soul that dwells in each human being and the personal consciousness is not possible without the help of Grace. That door must be opened by pure Grace!

After having these profound personal experiences, I started to study the ancient scriptures in order to understand from the intellectual point of view how to better incorporate the teachings.

For ever and ever, I will be grateful to Baba for answering all my questions. This is what a real Guru is all about. You trust Him and He gives Himself to you. Totally, no less. This is an unbelievable, evident fact! This is what shaktipat is all about. The Grace of understanding, of growing, of becoming a new being, of actualizing a hidden potential, of overcoming a life-time of hidden suffering, of finding answers to the most private concealed questions without the need, or the ability of expressing them in words.

Baba Muktananda is all for me. My spiritual father, my brother, my friend; my hope for the moment of death, my daily companion at every moment. His blessings continued to manifest during my life-time in uncountable circumstances. I trust His advice in everything, He is close-by and fully alive for me here and everywhere. His wisdom is incomparable. The more I read his words, the deeper the meanings appear to my understanding. An unending process of discovery, growth, and wonder takes place on a daily basis. The goals of a healthy, creative, productive life are being constantly fulfilled.

From His teaching I could clearly see that a human life lived only for the body, in the body, to please the body, is a tragic denial of the power of life itself. The river of humanity being dragged inevitably into the vortex showed me the tragedy underlining the times of war. This is what war is all about, a whirlpool for the destruction of bodies living only in the body, of flesh devoid of true human meaning; of humans who believed that the petty activities related to the physical body are all there is in human life.

We were all transported into the hurricane of despair, depression, powerlessness, and desolation, after twenty years of dictatorship all over Europe. Some lost their lives and some, like myself continued to live with the open wound of grief, without understanding why and what happened.

Finally, Baba Muktanadas' teachings permitted me to overcome the old feelings and a clear reality of renewal pervaded all my life since then.

This is a poem that I wrote at that time:

BABA
Baba is a concrete manifestation
of The Divine Cosmic Mind.

By looking through Him,
my Soul can be illuminated
by the Pure True Light.

Baba is a window open
to the vision of perfect Beauty.

Baba is a transparent opening,
in the frame of relative space-time,
through which the Power, the Love
and the intense shining of the Cosmic Mind
can touch my Soul.

His loving gesture keeps the window open and transparent,
for my Soul to enjoy and to grow in happiness and in glory.

Baba is both the Wisdom and the Understanding
guarding the Point of Splendour that is the Indivisible One,
the Centre of the Vortex,
the Eternal Light and the real Self of All.

The Infinite Eternal Being,
the Cosmic Consciousness,
the All Pervasive Intelligence,
is The Mother of All,
loving, nurturing and friendly to all Its children.

Baba is a symbol; the Rose is a symbol;
the helper, the mean, the transition, and the transformation;

the Path, the Tao that we must follow
to reach beyond the brain,
with the help of the trained brain,
with attention, devotion,
concentrations and intensity of Will and Love.

The next year I returned to the Ashram in India for six months and in the following years I attended the Ashrams of New York and of Atlanta on several occasions.

I positively was becoming a different person. Radiant, full of Love and benevolence and with the inner certainty that some day I would attain the Goal.

The teachings of my Guru and Siddha Yoga Master

Gurudev Swami Muktananda Paramahamsa is my Guru. What is a Guru? In Sanskrit, the word means: Gu=darkness; Ru=Light; it defines an advanced individual who can dispel the darkness in his/her disciples and provide Light for their awakening. A real, highly developed individual who is a Guru is extremely rare. It requires a life-time of purification and dedication, together with a profound understanding of Cosmic and Human Nature. Most important, her/his *'intentions'* must be totally selfless and fully offered to the Superior Self.

A True Guru is the physical representation of the Higher Self of All. It is an absolutely pure incarnated Being that serves as a clear window for the flowing of Subtle Energies that are not material, but very subtle and are called 'spiritual'.

In the tradition of my Guru and, therefore, in my tradition, a child recognizes the 'Call' very early in life, preserves her/his celibacy and chooses the path of selfless service in order to be able to obtain a total purification of the physical body. This comes about through years and years of study, devotion, and dedication. But, it will never be complete until the seeker finds his/her own Guru from whom the Grace must be received and given.

What is Grace in this context? It is the giving and taking of Spiritual, Unconditional, and Divine Love. It is the sanctification and final purification of the individual aspirant with the Blessings of his/her own Guru. It is "giving and taking" because the desire for total "Liberation" must be so strong in the seeker that she/he approaches the Guru with the intention of actively "stealing" the Grace, not only of "passively" receiving It. If the seeker is ready, the desire will be very strong and the already purified body will be an empty vessel ready to be filled with Grace. Then, the mysterious event called "Liberation" will certainly occur.

A true Guru is an extremely rare and blessed Being. To find one, recognize Her/Him, and obtain His/Her Blessings, is a very rare event in one life. To take advantage of the Blessings requires years of study, practice, and selfless dedication. But, the reward is the fulfillment of one's most Sacred Desire, for ever.

The main teachings of Gurudev Swami Muktananda for beginners were very simple in appearance: "God dwells in you, as you"; "See God in each other." It takes patience and lots of meditation to really understand what it means that God dwells in you, as you. It is not so simple, it involves a complete new cosmic concept to be assimilated and visualized. If the Infinite Being dwells in me, as me, it means that this apparent body and the little personal 'ego' are only a shell!.

At the beginning I learned that I am not the body. I am not this person that appears to be real. This person is a Temple for the manifesting Eternal Existence. We can cope with our mundane life applying concentration, discipline, and great devotion. Then, the freedom and happiness that are naturally inside us will bubble up and pervade our mundane self. This will permit us to cross the ocean of sorrow untouched and in serenity.

I started to learn to control my thoughts. During meditation the brain will continue to produce thoughts and the beginner is confused by these activities of the brain. Gurudev Muktananda advised us to be detached, to let the thoughts come and not pay attention to them. Instead, repeat the mantra.

Achieve mental and spiritual peace. Accept oneself as Divine, have compassion of our' and others' ignorance and maintain a state of contentment.

One of the main teachings that I learned from my Guru is about the pure love that springs from the heart.

Love from the core of our being is serene, generous, vast, and all inclusive recognizing both the limitations and the divinity of all beings.

Love from our centre is sincere, kind, not attached, benevolent, tolerant, but not blind. It applies some restrictions rather on itself than on others.

Love from the centre is able to perceive, judge and discriminate based on apparent characteristics of people, but these aspects are seen as superficial and do not affect the depth of love itself, only its responses.

Love from our centre is both objective and subjective. It is objective in the sense that it is based on true freedom, it transcends all personal aspects, is not binding, it trusts and openly offers itself. It is subjective in the sense that it is a deep, intimate joy, everlasting as a permanent inner condition, not as a transitory fluctuating wave.

Love from the centre does not imply any action. It is a being and not a becoming. Nevertheless, it may be a guiding principle for action. It is the healing of all fears, the support of all doubts, the balsam on all wounds, the hope in all despairs, the eternal in all impermanent, the new beginning at every end.

Love from the core of ourselves gives courage, self esteem, and independence. Love from the centre is simple, modest, unimposing, discrete, faithful, persistent, and dedicated. It may try to help by offering only a vague suggestion, or may be the solid strong hand pulling the victim our of the pit. It has no expectations and is not based on any exchange.

Love from the centre is in touch with the deep essence of all living creatures and also with the more apparent personal core of each.

Love from the centre is also called "Unconditional Love," the "Divine-All-Inclusive-Benevolence that sees no differences."

Baba would also talk about the most ancient Sanskrit expression, in Vedic terms: *SatChitAnanda.*

"Sat" has a very vast meaning, indicating 'That which Is', or 'Exist'. The Essence of Being. Not a personal being, or a personal god, but the Pure Subtle Essence of Existence.

"Chit" is the subtlest aspect of conscious intelligence. "Chit" is all pervasive, *non-relational*-intelligent-consciousness, before manifesting in the world. When it manifests, It is named *"Chiti"* and is concealed by the veils of manifestation.

"Ananda" is the Bliss of Perfection.

So, the Sanskrit expression *SatChitAnanda* can be briefly translated: *"Existence, Intelligent-Awareness, Joy-of-Perfection".* These are not *attributes* of the Divinity, or something superimposed.
They Are The Divine Self.

I will now try to explain these terms.

In our Western culture we consider always the word 'consciousness' as being 'relational'. We mean that *'one subject is aware of an object'* and that this *awareness* is somehow related to the function of a physical organ called *the brain*. This is not what 'cosmic consciousness' means in Sanskrit.

The ancient Vedic Seers realized that the universe is a web of relationships. In order for 'everything' to be related to 'everything else' there must be some 'form of information-processing' (expressing the concept in modern terms).

For this to take place, the underlying essential elements are, using modern terminology: *intelligent planning and knowledge= Cosmic Consciousness= The Mind of God (in Western terms)=Dynamic Evolution.*

This All Pervasive Cosmic Intelligence is the intrinsic Essence of everything. But, not 'everything' is conscious of it.

Many humans are not conscious of their own real essence because they are constantly distracted by external events and they don't know who, or what, they are.

The real essence of Life manifests as Order and Organization. The Universal Laws rule the most intimate processes of chemical and biological interactions, both inside our human body and in the Universe at large.

For example, the process of photosynthesis is very complex and is the fundamental condition for our planet to sustain Life. It could not "happen just by chance alone" as some scientists like to say. [1]

Another example is the exact behaviour of the genetic material called DNA and RNA responsible for the structural manifestation of all living forms across millennia of evolution.

More examples are provided by the specific interaction of enzymes and hormones at the cellular level of all living creatures.

These are only some examples out of many, but we can say with entire certainty that the Vast Universe, our Solar system included, is not the product of blind chance.

---

1   Foot-note: In scientific terms, the word 'chance' is a statistical expression; it is linked to the rules of mathematical 'probability' and used to express the results of biological studies. The living cell or organism cannot be studied without killing it; this means: freezing a condition in time. Life is dynamic and cannot be studied directly. Therefore, the results of investigations are always expressed as 'probabilities'. The word 'chance' means only that the probabilities of something to happen are low 'when studied in the lab'. Real Life cannot be reduced to lab. experiments eliminating all 'variables' and 'errors'. The expression: 'by chance' should be restricted to technical lab. research.

This fact was clear to ancient Sages who declared that the Universe is based on: Sat = existence; Chit = intelligent-non-relational-consciousness; Ananda= bliss of perfection.

When our brain it is properly trained by years of study and application, it becomes able to connect with some aspects of the Free-Intelligent-Cosmic-Consciousness. The so called human '*intelligence*' is *not* located *inside* our biological brain!

Human intelligence is not 'an accidental by-product of matter' as materialists like to say.

We become intelligent the moment in which our grey matter becomes able to establish a connection with the All-pervasive-cosmic-intelligence.

Our physical shell is only a shell, at all levels.

The Consciousness filling the shell, constantly encourages the establishment of contacts between a truly Self-Conscious Human Being and the All-pervasive-intelligence. The degree of human intelligence depends from the structure and complexity of the connections that have been achieved.

An easy example can be given by comparing our biological grey matter with a "*wave-sensitive-device.*" In the same way as we tune our radio to a far away transmitting station and we obtain the information emitted by the station, so, the same happens with our brain. The training of our brain through years of study is meant to create conditions that permit the reception of the type of waves in which we are interested.

The Cosmic Consciousness is never separated from His own Manifestation. It has a transcendent and an immanent aspect.

This concept is especially difficult for Western people, who are used to think on God as being a person. If God is an old man, or an anthropomorphic being, it is almost impossible to understand the concepts of being transcendent. The moment we grow into the knowledge of a truly Subtle-Spiritual-Universe, we may start to expand our consciousness and liberate ourselves from the oppression of matter.

The Transcendent aspect of the Divine is the pure potential aspect, unknown to us, as we don't have the capacity of perceiving extremely subtle non-material vibrations.

The Immanent aspect is all the universe that we perceive, including ourselves. All is "God" inside and out side, everywhere.

"You perceive the world depending on your degree of knowledge or igno-rance. The world is as you see it!" used to say Shree Swami Muktananda.

When the student of Siddha Yoga becomes immersed in this knowledge, he perceives the inner and the outer world as a vibration of Consciousness. Every work and activity becomes full of joy with perfect identification with the Divine.

Baba Muktananda did not try to impose any specific world view. He encouraged his students to become perfect Beings in order to obtain that sublime state in which you know that you are not dominated by any particular element. You are totally free, merging in the Divine Vibrations.

"There is nothing to renounce or to seek," would say Baba,
"You, yourself, Are the Play of Universal Consciousness!
You create, maintain, destroy, conceal yourself, and bestow Grace!
Recognize who and what you really are!
There is no need to repudiate the world, only get rid of the constric-tions caused by lack of awareness!"

The ignorant is kept in darkness because of three major obstacles, or constrictions:
'*Anava Mala*', the conviction of being *separated* from the DivineSource, feeling alone, abandoned, unconnected with everything else.
'*Mayiya Mala*' the perception of *differences,* the feeling of help-lessness, of depression, of being a victim, unable to cope and to overcome.
'*Karma Mala*' the belief of being the *performer* of actions (selfish ego), pride, arrogance, possessiveness, conceit, and egotism.

The study and understanding of these teachings, meditations, chanting, scrip-tures and mantra repetitions, help gradually to overcome ignorance. The goal is to reach the inner, personal, convincing 'Certainty', derived from the experience inside oneself, of the uninterrupted, constant and permanent presence of the Divine Vibration of Perfection in all events and actions of one's daily life.

We don't have to believe in any dogma, or in any compulsory statement, we only need to be calm, observe the subtle working of natural Laws around us, study the process, and try to avoid the constant useless chatting of the non-trained human brain.

Then, gradually, we will start relaxing the stress, the tension, the fear, the need to impose our ego on others, and our constant deep insecurity.

By repeating silently inside ourselves some words having beautiful meanings, such as Devotion, Beauty, Compassion and trying to capture their deep value, we focus on subtle energies that will give us an experience of inner peace and tranquility.

Baba Muktananda also insisted that we maintain mentally the company of Saints. He would say:

"Read the poetry of Saints, read the Scriptures, repeat the Mantra!"

All these methods would help reducing the useless activity of the brain and focus on who we really are.

At the Ashram we used to do Hata-yoga every morning and then we would study scriptures and texts helping our meditation.

For me, the most important and healing experiences were the long hours of chanting. People who have not experienced the incredible cheering effect of long chanting, may say that such practice is boring and is a form of self hypnosis. Well, unfortunately there is a lot of ignorance about what we have never experienced. But, the truth is that the greatest therapeutic effect of the life in the Ashram is the time dedicated to chanting.

The body and the brain become so happy of expressing love and more love, repeated many, many times, that they become Love itself! When the Chant is over, you feel the vibrations for long time inside the head and the body. Every cell becomes attuned, they all function in great harmony and a supreme joy emerges from this physiological well-being.

The first time that I visited the Ashram in Ganeshpuri, I could not chant because my voice would not come out. Years of stress had tightly locked my vocal cord. It is unbelievable how long it takes to release that stress. I started to chant whispering; the voice would come out only from the throat, not from the chest. You may scream and yell, but that is also from the throat out.

On the contrary, the true chanting is deep from the chest and involves all your respiratory system. You push the diaphragm down, inhale deeply into the belly, and from there the sonority of the voice arises. It is quite a different involvement of circulatory, respiratory, and internal organs system! It is a wonderful experience, but it needs time, patience, and dedication, as everything else!

In my house, where I live now, many, many years later, I still follow somehow the routine and the ritual of the Ashram. I never completely stopped the practice of deep breathing exercises, meditation and chanting; always remembering the joy and the devotion that bring serenity and beauty to our lives.

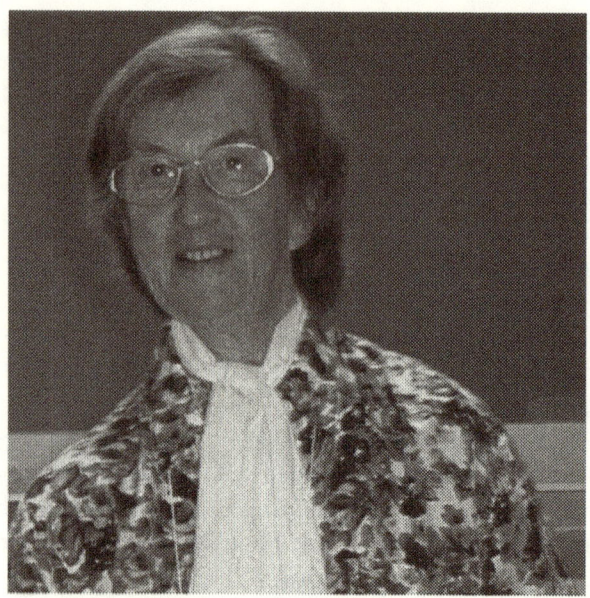

Picture of the Author

Times of war:
Out of Venezuela and resident in Canada

Events and conditions drive us toward
Change and adaptation; we must learn and
constantly tread a new path.

Economical and political crisis in South America.

In the early 1980s the political landscape in Venezuela and in general in all South America, became more and more confused and uncertain. The oil concessions to the foreign company in the west of the country expired around 1983. Decline in oil production and a major political convulsion accompanied this period. Poverty increased dramatically and street violence, kidnappings, and insecurity were everywhere. No viable solutions for the social problems of health, education, and labour organization were implemented.

I realized that the general climate of the country was not what I desired for my children. During street demonstrations against the Government more than twenty students had been shot by the police during one academic year. I did not want my children to get involved in riots, but if they became university students they would have to participate in the general protest as everybody else.

During 1982 I sold all my investments in real estate in Caracas.

Shortly after, the value of the local currency, the Bolivar, fell from Bolivares 4,50 for one US Dollar, to Bs. 20.00 for one US Dollar.

Just a short time later, the change was Bs. 600.00 for one US Dollar. The crisis became terrible.

Divorce and new residence in Canada with my sons

I talked with my husband and decided to move to Canada with the children. He decided to stay and take care of his business.

We had a short, friendly divorce. Shortly after I was happy to learn that he had married a good friend of mine, a good lady who took care of him until his death, several years later.

My mother was very sick and passed away in 1985.

All the conditions were set for me to move out of South America for good, after thirty-eight years of intense activity and success. The finger of Destiny was pointing very clearly toward Canada, where I had studied and worked as a Resident in the late 1950s.

I remembered the time when I had left Italy for good. You need courage and trust in yourself and in God's help! Just let go of everything, grab a suitcase and go!

I was sixty; it was a good time to retire from the stressful academic and gynaecological work.

I had the responsibility of two teenagers, but the positive aspect was that my older son would be accepted as a student by Mc Gill University in Montreal, after he passed his English test. He did pass, and we all happily moved to Quebec, as new Canadian Residents.

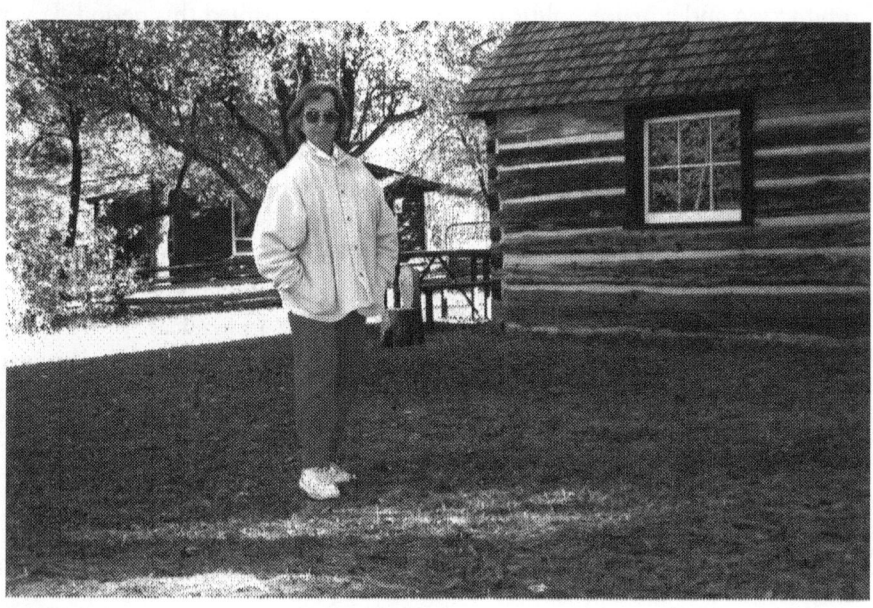

Fourth Part:

My learning and self discovery

*In the Friendly, Imposing Giant of the
Great North, Nature is Vast and Pure,
A Safe Haven of Peace and Serenity*

Times of Peace:
Dedication to my personal evolution

The old story of my first encounter with Canada

Since I first visited Canada to study at the University of Toronto, in 1958-60, I fell in love with the beauty of the lakes and forests of northern Ontario. I used to spend my summer vacations there and go cross-country and downhill skiing in winter in my days off-duties.

The story of how I got the opportunity to first visit Toronto in 1958 is very curious. I received an invitation to visit Toronto while traveling in an airplane from Milan to Switzerland! A young couple sitting at my side in the airplane invited me! They asked me to spend the next Christmas vacation at their house in Ontario. This is how it all happened.

It was the fall of 1958 and we were flying from Milan, Italy, to Switzerland to go downhill skiing there. They were a nice young Canadian couple traveling as tourists in Europe. They were sitting beside me in the plane and we started to talk. At that time I had almost completed my post doctoral training in Italy, but I was very worried about my surgical skills. As they were very nice people, I opened my heart to them. My training period at the university of Milan would soon come to an end and I would become a "Specialist in Obstetrics and Gynaecology", but I had not been allowed any surgical training because the director of the Institution said that "surgery in not for women".

In Italy at that time, the position of women was very sad. They were just good for service, nothing else. At the hospital I was the only woman in a surgical specialty. I had to put up a big fight to be allowed in the "Doctors" lunch cafeteria, because, being a woman, I was supposed to go to the nurse's cafeteria. I won that fight and took my lunches at the doctors' cafeteria, but I did not win the one for the surgical training.

When I explained this situation to the Canadians, they found the whole story very funny and said:

"Come to Toronto for Christmas and we take you to Women's College Hospital, you may talk to them and see if they can accept you for training."

My eyes got wide open and my heart too.

"Yes! I certainly accept your invitation!", I said.

So, on December 20, 1958, with a little bag for a two-week vacation, I landed in Toronto at the house of my new friends. We had a good time for Christmas at their club and a couple of days later we finally went to visit the Woman's College Hospital.

In the large hall I saw on the left a big door with a sign "Human Resources-Secretary." My friends said,

"There it is, go in and talk."

My heart was beating hard ... what a moment!

I knocked at the door and went in.

The elegant young lady at the desk smiled and asked,

"How can I help you?"

With uncertain voice, I explained that I was an Italian doctor and a specialist in Gynaecology, but I had not received the proper surgical training, as it was refused to women in Italy.

She thought it was a good joke and laughed at it.

But, I was dam serious. She said,

"So, what is it that you want?"

"Surgical training!" I said.

"Well, you are very lucky," she said, "Because the Hospital needs you! We have an opening in the Department of OBS-GYN starting January first. Do you want to take it? The salary is very small and you must live in the hospital as a Senior Intern Resident. Do you accept it?"

The emotion made me spin ...

"Yes, thank you!"

I was just able to whisper. Unbelievable ...!

But, very quickly it became tangible reality as the secretary prepared the contract, looked at my papers, and shortly after all was ready for me to sign.

Next, she warned me:

"As you are now employed, but you are presently on a tourist Visa, you must re-enter the Country as a Landed Immigrant. Nevertheless, we can wait for the tree months of probation; then, I will prepare your papers and you only need to drive to the US border and re-enter Canada."

Well, in half hour my life had turned upside down, or upside up!

I was now officially employed at the University of Toronto (as the Hospital was attached to the University) and would receive the surgical training I needed.

Thank you God! This is a miracle!

These two years, 1959-60, were wonderful and Canada remained in my heart.

Making a dream come true

We first came to Montreal in fall of 1984 for the registration of my son at Mc Gill University. I went back to Caracas as my mother was very sick and finally, I returned for good with my younger son in the spring of 85.

I bought a 100 acres-woods, and 30 acres-tillable, farm with an old, original, hundred years old log house in Glengarry County, near Alexandria. It was very close to the Quebec border, just one hour away from Montreal. My sons could easily make short visits and enjoy the open air.

All our ties with South America and the world remained as a good memory in our heart, but we had to face everything new.

The children succeeded at school and I learned to be a Canadian farmer. A big red tractor helped me seed 30 acres of alfalfa and I had a good yearly crop for the neighbour's horses.

The woods were a mystery and a refuge in the depth of mother earth.

The log house was another mystery of intimacy …

I started to feel very mystic and I resumed the Yoga practices that I used to do at the Ashram, in India.

Spiritual experiences started to happen.

Five intense years of Yoga Retreat in rural Ontario

I remained by myself at the farm for five years. My spiritual growth increased exponentially. It was joy, serenity, and the presence of the Divinity in every thing everywhere and in everyone.

During my long meditations, I experienced the awakening of all my chakras, as my Guru, Baba Muktananda had promised me, if I would persist in the practice. My main desire was for Peace, personal peace, peace for my children, peace for the world.

One day, a profound, loud voice told me in Spanish "Tendras Paz!"—You will have peace-And this promise became truth. The absolute certainty of the constant presence of Benevolent Cosmic Consciousness. No fear, no loneliness, no doubts, no uncertainties, but serenity, self-assurance, contentment and Peace!

The spiritual experiences became an everyday surprise and meditation was a natural way of being. I used to take long walks in the woods and be constantly in a state of contemplation and absorption in a wonderful dimension of beauty and serenity.

All what saints describe in their writings is absolutely true. But, it is our task to create the surroundings in which the different levels of subtle reality can become perceptible to a brain that is completely calm.

It is not necessary to "sit" in meditation, unless you are a very beginner, still at the stage of calming the confusion of thoughts. Every act, from collecting wood, to eating, to cleaning the little house, all can be acts dedicated to the company of Saints, to contemplate the sacred mantras, to discuss with your High Inner Self in complete freedom.

The breathing exercises were very important at the beginning of the day to open the channels of energy and purify the inner and outer bodies. Some Yoga stretching and asana made me feel really alive and full of vigour! Then a fast walk around a field of alfalfa increased my appetite for breakfast!

In the property, there was also a natural spring and a deep pond, but I dared to plunge in it only in warm summer days. The water came from deep inside the earth and was icy!

In the little log house there was a good steel fireplace and the big job every year was to decide which trees to fell for the next year heating. That was an ongoing task for my children when they came to visit. Then, they would cut the logs and in August each years (when there are no mosquitoes, or black flies), the big red tractor would help me carry the logs to storage to dry. That task was so new and unusual for us that I needed many advices from neighbours to properly understand the handling of the fireplace.

Nevertheless, I had two chimney fires in the five years! Not a very good record! But no real damage, beside a big scare! Now, I know everything about 'creosote' building up inside the chimney!

I did not want to have animals because they require attention and are a distraction, but in that old setting it was inevitable to have cats, otherwise the number of mice would grow exponentially and they would eat my food and also me! So, I ended up with tenth of cats, all wild, but very useful!

The sources for the day long meditation were the scriptures that I studied. Gurudev's most important teachings were related to the capacity of deeply and sincerely *recognize who and what you really are.* In order to introduce us to this concept Baba Muktananda would tell the story of the baby lion.

> *"A poor farmer found an abandoned baby lion and raised it as a pet. The farmer had two donkeys to help him plough his little field and the baby lion actually believed to be a baby donkey and that his destiny was to be working ploughing the soil. Only when he grew up and met a real lion, he was told that he was a lion and not a slave donkey! This knowledge set him free!"*

The understanding that we are not the body, but Intelligent-Cosmic-Consciousness, will set us free! We expand our awareness by eliminating petty concerns, useless worries and instead, filling the mind with the feeling of being alive, full of joy and in touch with all of nature. Every activity is dedicated to the discovery of beauty, of perfection in all aspects of our environment.

"The world is as you see it!"

How true! Every day I would understand this statement more and more deeply. All contacts with the 'Media' were cut completely; until today, I have no links with news, information, and what happens in the world; no radio, no newspapers, no television. I don't need to be informed about none of these things. On the contrary I need to deeply heal myself and become a pure mirror of the Divine Perfection. This is my real task: becoming aware that I am a free lion and not a slave donkey!

I worked daily on setting free my inner energy, on circulating the subtle force related to the chakras. I could sense how my body would respond every day with greater joy. The Yoga teachings of Shree Baba Muktananda were very precise and easy to follow with concentration and patience. The awakening and purification of the spiritual channels of energy gradually merge the awareness of the personal self with the transcendent beauty of the Self of All.

Practice and self-analysis: *the three 'malas'*

First consideration: Why did I suffer for so many years from post-traumatic stress disorder? The medical diagnosis relates this condition to the persistence of war's bad memories.

But, the reality was that *I was feeling separated from God.* This, according to my Guru's teachings, is the first *mala: anava-mala.* It is the belief of being alone, separated from the source of Life and of Love.

When I was a child, the teachings of Adeline and of Anna, the story of Jesus and the statue of the Sheppard in the school chapel, helped me connect with God and with the source of Love.

Later, the horrors of war raised doubts about the *goodness of creation.* I suspected that all was a lie and that the benevolent being did not exist at all. The entire universe collapsed around me and only ruins were left. I repressed in my subconscious this unbearable uncertainty and went on with my studies and my life. But, the real problem was not solved. The real problem was between my Soul and my God, inside myself. The scholar and professional activities were only a welcome distraction, outside my real Self.

This psychological condition of restrained anger and anxiety produced a serious imbalance in my metabolism that manifested twenty years later in an invasive cancer of the thyroid.

If at that time I would have known what I know today about *preventive holistic care and preventive medicine that can be achieved by balancing subtle energies,* I would have probably used the acupuncture and acupressure techniques to keep the balance of my biological system. But, the Chinese medical science started to be popular in the West only much later.

Second consideration: The clinical death sentence and the subtle intuition that guided my recovery.

When I was doing the meditations on my own death, I discovered that after my passing away, every thing would be apparently the same.

Therefore, my life had no value. But, something inside me strongly reacted and claimed that the life of every manifestation has an intrinsic value. If this were not so, then suicide would be an easy and simple solution for all difficulties in life.

The life of every manifestation has a value because all is interconnected. One's own life is not a private property; it is shared with the entire universe. Every manifestation can always chose to perform a task that is useful for others. This is precisely the difference. One may only experience fear of death and a selfish desire to keep enjoying life.

Or, there may be a desire to enjoy life and also a selfless desire of being useful to others.

This is a very subtle difference of perception and an important moment of evolution. If we say: I am separated from God, this is *Anava Mala,* but if we also say I am insignificant and worthless, this is *Mayiya Mala,* the second of our wrong beliefs. The concept that "I AM important and significant" may be wrongly interpreted as a self-enhancement of the little selfish ego. But, in the case of a dawning awareness of a—*selfless usefulness*-, it is the emergence of a new awareness of the superior Self, the real I AM, that shines forth for the first time.

This meant that, while doing my death meditations, I had a sudden realization that I was not necessarily just an insignificant selfish ego; but that I was a real I AM, in the higher meaning of the expression.

My manifested individuality was meaningful in a cosmic sense.

I had been useful to others and I could continue to do so, if I survived that test. The entire meaning of my life changed focus during those meditations. The social and professional training that I had received had instructed me to do the best I could in my own personal interest. The concept of being a doctor "to help others" was certainly not dominant in the academia!

That subtle difference in the perception of my goal in life permitted me to overcome the ignorance related to *mayiya mala*. A big evolutionary step!

Third consideration: this is related to the concept of *being the doer*.

In Sanskrit terms it is called *Karma mala*. Every selfish action, every deed performed for benefiting the little ego, will bring about some Karma. On the contrary, if all mundane activity is offered to the Supreme, no Karma derives from the daily performance of duties.

This subtle difference in the intention behind every act was for me very difficult to grasp. Until I went to India I could not really understand the meaning of this statement. In my life in the hospitals or in my professional performance anywhere, things had to be done, because they had to be done and most of the times it was an emergency. So, there was no specific awareness of any intention, but just acting according to well established clinical routines and methods. This is our usual behaviour in the West, we are strictly pragmatic and often act as robot. Precisely, this is the mistake and the aspect of being 'asleep' and not 'awaken'.

When we are fully awaken, we have the constant realization that we are co-creators with the Cosmic Consciousness in every thing we do.

We do not follow any more a blind hospital routine in order not to receive reprimands from the boss; we do not work only to keep one's pay-cheque coming in every month. The intention behind every act is different; it is an offering to Life and to Divine-Manifestation. No one needs to know, nobody needs to notice, but the whole individual performs with a stamina that is intimate and transcendent. The source of the renewed energy proceeds from higher level of Consciousness.

By being attuned with the Cosmic, the individual's will power is enhanced because it is in harmony with the Whole.

The free will is still present and we may make serious mistakes and momentarily loose our connection. We are still fully human and every step can be a progress or a regression; but, if we are sincere, we will be able to correct our errors and return to the Divine At-one-ment.

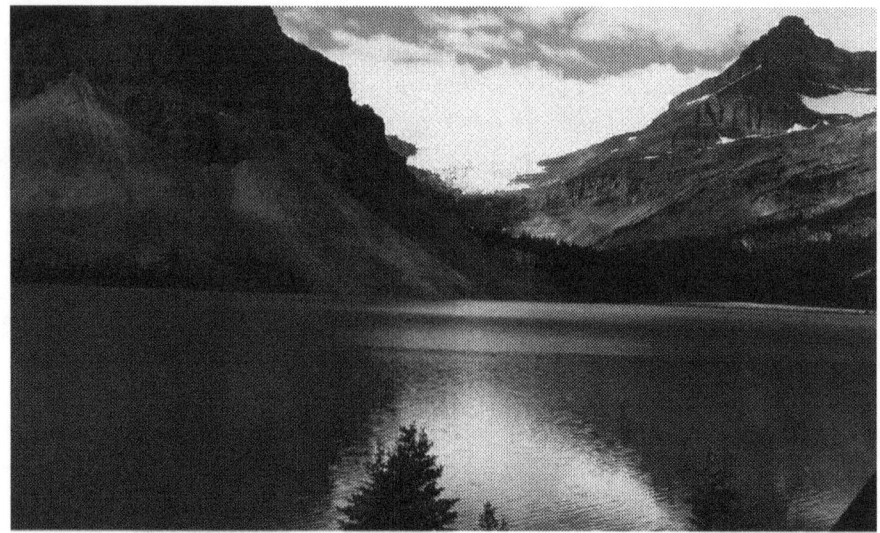

Glacier and lake in the Canadian Rockies

A few guidelines for our development

First, we want to fully understand the meaning of certain words. These are:

Wisdom
Understanding
Benevolence
Severity
Beauty
Devotion
Clear intelligence

I borrowed these very significant expressions from the 'Tree of Life' and tried to disclose a possible 'return Path', from the dense manifestation to the subtle spiritual vibrations:

Clear intelligence

The first task is the management of the confusing thoughts; the working of the brain must be under the control of the person and not the opposite. Most people are unable to control their brain and become slaves of recurring emotions, anxiety, and negative feelings. No progress can be achieved until this condition persists. Start by looking in the dictionary and find all the meanings of the word "clear." Imagine something clear, like a recently cleaned window, clear water, clear crystal, and so on. Next, look in the dictionary the meaning of "intelligence." That is a bit more difficult; you may need also a book on normal psychology and one on neuroscience. The truth is that most authors do not agree on the meaning of the word *intelligence*. So, there you have work to do. You must create a significant meaning for your personal intelligence. What does it mean for you to have a *clear intelligence*? When you have it, you will certainly know! No doubts or confusion will be left hanging around! Just clear skies! Remember that intelligence is not just an 'epi-phenomenon' of matter as materialists say!

Devotion

You cannot progress any further unless you posses a clear intelligence, given that the next task is Devotion. I visualize devotion, as the constant attention that a good mother gives to her newborn baby. So, if you want to develop dedication, or devotion, you must visualize your goal with clear intelligence. It could be some type of study, or activity, or anything that you desire intensely and that is supposed to fulfill your most cherished aspirations.

Devotion to something involves a serious decision. You must search and search; what are you really interested in; what makes you kick. You can read books about the great discoverer, for example in science, or in geography. People who dared to go where no one had gone before. Real heroes with a vision. You don't need to be a hero, but you most certainly have something that *really is of interest to you!* There is so much to search!

Beauty

Again look in the dictionary the several meanings of Beauty. A Greek temple has an imposing beauty; a calm lake has a special beauty; the smile of a child is beautiful. The best solution is to write down all the beautiful things you can think of. By doing this exercise during several weeks, you attain the goal of focusing the thoughts on a beautiful goal, enhancing your positive emotions and maybe finding what is really beautiful for you! As you walk and move around, find beauty everywhere! Find harmony!

Here you make a pause. These first three tasks should take you at least three months to stabilize your thoughts and your desire. Think that your entire life may depend on what you decide during these first months. So, take your time, but constantly thing about your tasks. You may go shopping and talk to others but in the back of your mind you continue to work on the three tasks.

Nevertheless, this period must come to an end. You must reach a reasonable decision that depends only on you. Do not talk to others about these tasks, they must be your private secret. Consult with encyclopaedias, and with serious texts, but don't chatter with others about the most important decision that you are ever going to take in your life. Remember that the decision is about *who you want to be!*

Severity

Here comes the first important test. You must ask yourself: "Am I serious about my goals?" Look at yourself in the mirror and answer the question. Then, again get your dictionary and write down all the meanings of the word severity.

It can be a long list. Sometimes severity is unpleasant, but it is absolutely necessary toward yourself. Do not mix other people or the memory of a though teacher. No! severity toward yourself means *sincerity*. Sincerity in the depth of your heart. You don't want to be a superficial butterfly following the rules of he latest fashion. You want to be your real, deep, sincere, innocent, good, own self.

Benevolence

This is the balance with severity. You must be able to forgive yourself and others. Remember well: everybody and everything must be fully forgiven from the very bottom of you heart, before you can progress any further. Forgiveness toward yourself is the first step. We all have been impatient, nasty, or unfair with some one; we all have had some uncomfortable shakings in some opportunities; we have resentments, sense of injustice; jealousy and so on. Let all the dirt come up to the surface; be fully conscious of all the details and then, with great benevolence, let them all go for ever!

The question was asked: do we have to forgive also the very bad people. The answer is:

> *"It is not you who forgive! You are never the doer! The Divinity in you is the real doer. Your task is to be fully conscious, to participate*

with good will in the process. Do not resist the flow of the Way! The Flow of the Superior Will! Be humble and understand that it is your task to dominate the little proud ego! The little ego is the one who want to resist. Surrender to the Superior Self inside you; forgive all, also the very bad ones. It is never your task to judge anyone!"

Understanding

The meaning of life, of ourselves, of others, is a mystery that we try to unravel. We need to be humble, to stand-under, to shut up our little ego, our selfishness, and our desire to criticize. In order to understand, we must work with our Right brain. The *meanings of Life* are abstract symbols most of the times. For example, mathematics and chemistry, are essential parts of science, but their meanings are abstract. In the same way, the deep meaning of events sometime escapes us and we do not understand why something happened the way it did.

We need concentration, reflection, visualization, and a deep, objective analysis, in order to grasp the significance of certain events and of certain people. A superficial, ego-centred look does not let us perceive the truth behind appearances. The process of Understanding is a long, and patient practice, that must be taken very seriously, or we will pass through life without understanding anything!

Wisdom

The end result of our effort to reach perfection will be coronate when we obtain wisdom! When you reach this point, you are very advanced, you have worked seriously for months or years to clarify, overcome, and develop patience and clarity. What is Wisdom? It is the complete *Intuition* of the *Big Picture,* of the whole. Consult the best dictionaries and write in your notebook all the associations that you can find. In order to help your imagination. Let me give you an esoteric definition:

Wisdom is the Light that gives Light to the Stars.

Does this sound wonderful? In spiritual terms it is almost impossible to define true Wisdom, because it is the inner Vision of the All, as the only supreme Reality.

Together with the study of the meaning of certain words, it is useful to become familiar with different concepts related to the attributes of the universe. The following is a summary of these notions.

Attributes of the Universe.

The first attribute of the Universe is Existence.

This universe "exists." [Don't ask 'why' because such question can be answered only in the sense of cycles] The fact is that this universe exists. Even if, in a certain sense, it is an illusion, this does not deny its existence. In terms of quantum physics, some aspects are illusion, in terms of relativity, other aspects are illusions. In terms of the ancient Eastern philosophy of Vedanta, most of it is only appearances and illusions. Nevertheless, for us manifested beings, this universe exists, and we exist in it and with it.

The second attribute of the universe is Intelligence.

Intelligence is not an 'epi-phenomenon-of matter' as certain materialists would like to believe. The Universe is itself Intelligence and Order.

There are well recognized Universal Laws that coordinate the relationships of all the multiple aspects in an orderly fashion. So, this universe exists and is organized by Intelligent Laws of Order and Harmony. The practical examples of intelligent organization can be found in basic biochemical behaviour of genetic material (e.g. DNA, RNA); in the biochemistry of photosynthesis; in the coordination of the nervous systems; in the precise functioning of enzymes and hormones and in many other features of life and cosmic characteristics.

The third attribute of the Universe is it Manifestation.

This Manifestation takes place at infinite levels of subtlety. The subtlest aspects are impossible for humans to imagine because they are not material. They are what we call "Divine," for lack of another word. This is the word that humans use, in order to define something that cannot be named otherwise. This Divine aspect of the Universe is all pervasive, as are all Its Laws. Nothing can escape the Universal Divine Laws of Order and Harmony.

Therefore, humans are part of the Divine Universal Laws. But, when humans are only inside the gross body, they cannot imagine the real meaning of these words. When they are able to expand the level of the gross consciousness and reach some intuition of a more subtle consciousness, humans recognize their true Universal Divine Nature.

Attributes of Humans

The first attribute is that they Exist.

Their subtle existence is inside an apparently gross cover of matter.

The gross cover of solid matter is in a certain sense an illusion. In terms of quantum physics it is certainly an illusion. In term of levels of vibrations it is also an illusion. Humans have at least four bodies of different densities and different attributes, but most humans ignore this fact. The illusion is supported by the fact that humans need to infuse energy into that gross matter. They must derive energy from the metabolism of products of the planet by eating food and water. They must derive energy from the Light of the Stars by breathing at least twenty times a minute. If humans do not provide energy to the gross matter of the body, the cover itself appears to be inert and unable of manifesting life. Therefore, the gross cover of matter is needed to have a tool that is adapted to the presence on this planet.

Nevertheless, in abstract reality, Human subtle existence has nothing to do with the gross matter cover. Human existence consists of different layers of subtle energy that are shared with the rest of the subtle energies of the universe. The gross matter cover is just a big illusion! If we remove that illusion we see a *Holographic Universe* reflected in a *Holographic Human brain!*

> *The so called 'Mind of God' is all there is everywhere.*
> *The only eternal, infinite existing Reality.*
> *The spiritual reality tells us that*
> *there is "No Man without God and no God without Man."*
> *Since ever and for ever we are ONE.*

A topic for profound meditation!

The second attribute of humans is Intelligence.

Humans are intelligent in their subtle aspect because they share the Divine Intelligent Universal Laws of Order and Harmony. But, their gross cover of matter is not intelligent in the same sense. It is not self-aware and does not consciously recognize the Divine Laws of Order and Harmony at the same subtle level. Therefore, those humans who believe that the gross cover of matter is their only real identity, cannot be truly intelligent and self-aware, because they lack communication with the subtle levels. They remain at the stage of sleeping beings, without intuition of the subtle intelligent levels. The problem deriving from remaining numb is that they are not aware of the concept of Order and Harmony that are attributes of the Divine Laws. They suffer greatly, create confusion, and are unable to understand and believe that the development of the faculty of intuition would allow them to function in better condition. They lack objective awareness and feel oppressed.

The third attribute of humans is Free Will to Manifest.

Both, the sleeping beings, or robots, enclosed inside the gross cover of matter and those humans who were able to develop intuition, possess Free Will to Manifest. Obviously, the types of manifestations of these two different kind of humans are very different.

Order and Harmony are the desire and intention of those developed into the awareness of the subtle energies.

The contrary conditions are promoted by the robots because of their permanent status at the gross level of solid matter constantly ruled by Fear and Aggression. This condition produces disorder, confusion, pain, and cruelty.

Because of the all-pervasiveness of the universal Divine Laws, the manifestations of Fear and Aggression produce laws of cause-and-effect that are very damaging for all humans and mostly for the robots themselves.

This explains why human thoughts are so powerful, both in the intention of following the Divine Laws and in the intention of not following them, and indulging in fear and aggression.

In conclusion, if humanity wants to reach a condition of Peace and universal Understanding, it must confront the heavy task of educating that part of humanity still at the sleeping stage.

They can easily learn that they are NOT the gross body of matter, but beautiful Divine Aspects of the Eternal Laws.

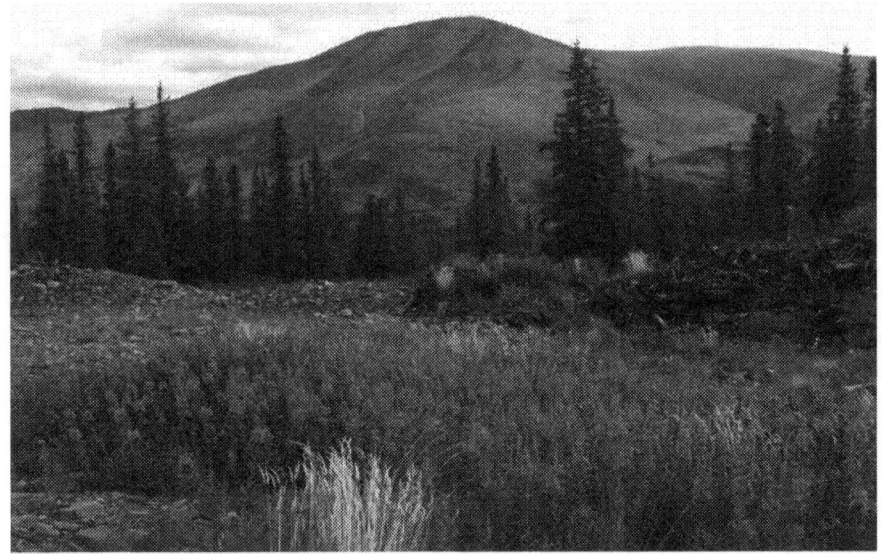

Flowers in the northern Tundra

Ancient definitions

Human powers (will, knowledge and action) and human qualities (subtle, egoistic and aggressive)

TABLE 1

Powers and Qualities

Powers	Qualities		
	Satvic	**Rajasic**	**Tamasic**
WILL	Beauty, Harmony Universal Love	Personal desires Egoistic intentions	Revengeful Aims Hatred against all
	Order, Growth	Selfish attachments	Destruction of all
	Perfection, All Good	Possessive passion	Negative intention
	Compassion for All	Accumulation greed	Cruelty, Sadism
KNOWLEDGE	Understanding	Ego-centred belief	Accusatory, Low
	Objective analysis	Limited, Chaotic	Suspicious, Envy
	Vast, Big Picture	Subjective ignorance	Distrusting, Intrigue
	Focused Synthesis	Unstable, Confused	Inertia, Instincts
	Correlated, Inclusive	Crisis, self-victimizing	Secret confabulations
ACTION	Serene, Impartial	Impulsive, Dramatic	Violent, Destructive
	Efficient, Orderly	Ineffective, Insecure	Insensitive, Obsessive
	Respectful, tranquil	Contradictory, Helpless	Cruel, Hateful
	Just, Balanced	Fearful, Sorrowful	Blind aggression
	Independent, Creative	Clinging, Oppressive	Deathly, Imposing
	~~	~~~~~~~~~~~~	~~~~~~~~~~~~
	VISION OF LIFE	EGO/VISION	VISION OF DEATH

Table 1.

No need of special explanations for this table. It is self-evident.

The three Human Qualities are related to degrees of personal evolution: higher, medium, and low (low evolution is always dominated by *fear and aggression*, the law of the jungle, to eat or to be eaten. It is the characteristic of dictators everywhere). The three Powers are common to everyone.

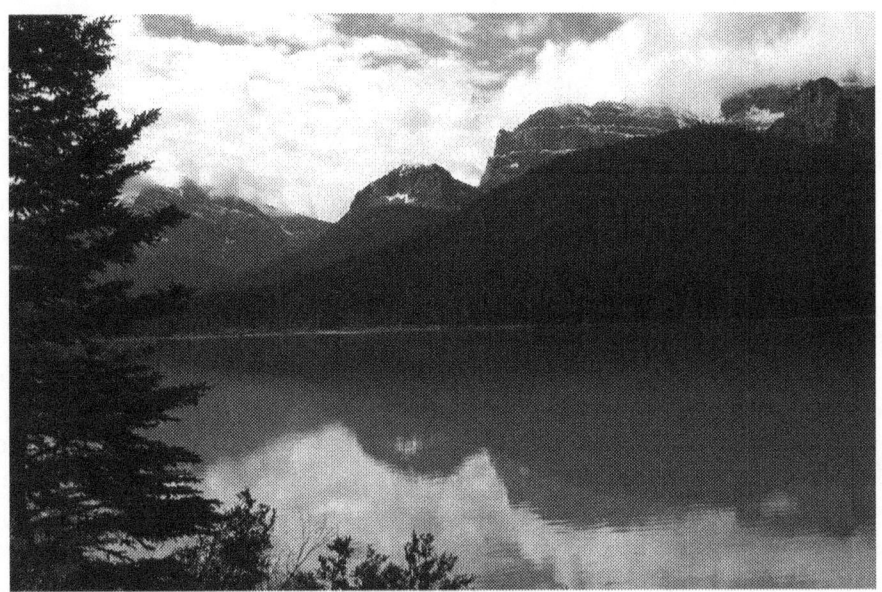

lake in The Canadian Rockies

The vision of the ONE

The ONE is Pure Light, Good, and Beauty. The ONE is outpouring Good and Beauty out of itself, as a great artist who expresses his/her sublime art. This outpouring manifests into the Divine Soul, also called the Self of All and into the Divine Cosmic Mind.

This is pure vibrant Light directly from the Source.

The so-called descent of Light is no real descent. It only implies that the frequency and intensity of the vibrations must be reduced in order to manifest at the level of what we call 'gross-matter'.

The One Divine Soul, the Self of All, absorbs lower vibrations.

The flashing forth of the Self of All at lower vibrations spreads into the 'atman' of each one of us (also called "soul personality").

The Reflection of the ONE, in the Self of All, becomes 'the many manifested souls'. These manifested personal souls have the goal of going through the experiences of life to purify the dense vibrations. Nevertheless, they don't loose the link of unity with the Universal Soul, the so-called Self of All, reflection of ONE.

The cycles of Manifestation and Re-absorption are constant and endless. The personal soul that was not able of purifying her/his vibrations, needs to re-incarnate in order to continue with the assigned task.

Other personal souls are able to achieve purification, and slowly progress on the path that will reunite them with the Source.

The expression 'purification' means: to be able of vibrating at higher frequencies, as compared with the low frequencies of 'matter.' In Table 1, the higher level of vibration corresponds to the Quality Satvic, in Sanskrit language.

Re-incarnation is the return of the personal soul to another cycle of purification; this is our work.

During the period of our manifested life, we have the subconscious '*memory*' of the outpouring of Goodness and Beauty that is the origin of ourselves, as ONE.

This '*memory*' is all around us and inside us, in the all-pervasive Divine Cosmic Mind. Its presence creates the longing that we experience for Good and for Beauty. Every human being desires Good and Beauty, because it is our common racial 'memory'. If we would not have that memory, very hidden inside us and very clear outside us, we would not have a clear consciousness of the opposites, that are: bad and ugly. We recognize the bad and the ugly, because we remember the Good and the Beautiful. The Self of All is always within each of us. Because of such Divine presence, we learn and we know.

We suffer because we are that manifested ONE, remembering His Joy of spreading Good and Beauty.

The dense vibrations that surround us need to be refined to complete the cycle of return.

Matter must be transformed into Light again.

Gross vibrations must be sublimated into "*unconditional love.*"

The Great Artist must wash his brushes and tools after He manifested His/Her sublime Art. We are here washing the tools.

TABLE 2.

	ONE PURE LIGHT GOOD BEAUTY SAT			
CHIT				ANANDA
DIVINE NOUS COSMIC MIND				**DIVINE SOUL SELF OF ALL**
Order-Life CONSCIOUSNESS				Essence PERFECTION
=================	Reduction MORE ==========	Of GROSS ==========	Vibrations VIBRATIONS ===========	==============
Slow process of	Manifested Atman/Manas Purification **Slow** MORE	Universe Prakriti Memory of **Return** SUBTLE	Intelligence Alma Mundi Good/Beauty **Path** VIBRATIONS	Suffering
Transformation	of	Matter	Into	Light

Explaining Table 2.

The Cosmic Infinite Eternity is dynamic energy constantly renovating itself in endless cycles. It is impossible for our little grey cells to capture the immensity of the transformations. Nevertheless, we could imagine the dynamic vortex as a cycle of returning energies transmuting themselves from very subtle vibrations into gross vibrations and then becoming very subtle again.

In Table 2., the un-manifest, extremely subtle, is called ONE.

In Sanskrit, three aspects are assumed: SAT, existence, CHIT, consciousness, ANANDA, bliss of perfection. The potentialities of Pure Light are Goodness and Beauty.

The intelligent manifested universe is composed of gradually more dense vibrations. The cyclic transformations involve a gradual return to subtle vibrations. Therefore, the complete cosmic cycles evolve from subtle vibrations, to gross vibrations and to subtle vibration again.

Humans may contribute to transmute matter into subtle energy by training the tool called '*brain*'. The human brain may learn to attune to spiritual thoughts and transmute dense vibrations into more subtle ones.

The well '*spiritually*' trained human brain may contribute to the cosmic process by functioning as the interface between gross matter and divine energy.

The practical consideration consists in controlling our thoughts.

What are we thinking all the time? What are the grey-cells chatting about? Are we vibrating with the joy of Goodness and Beauty? If we are not, then we could try to do so. Our senses perceive only Beauty, nothing else. We don't want to perceive anything else. Only Goodness and Beauty exist, only the ONE exists.

What is not Goodness and Beauty is produced by the low vibrations of insufficiently developed people.

We don't help at all by lowering our vibrations at their level.

We can certainly help by elevating our vibrations even more and be patient and wait until people develop.

Every human being is destined to evolve to perfection, sooner or later.

The whole human race is an important tool for Cosmic Evolution. No human will be left behind. The unique destiny of each of us is Goodness and Beauty. We may need thousands of repeated incarnations to understand this great truth, but there is no doubt that eventually we will '*understand.*'

In the scale of the so called '*return path*', we reach the level of 'understanding' just before we reach the wonderful level called '*wisdom.*' When we reach wisdom, we have accomplished our task. We have the satisfaction of being more than simple human beings. We have uncovered our spiritual Essence! Joy and Perfection unending!

There appear to be a large number of under-developed human beings because of the infinite grandiosity of the Cosmic Cycles, from our limited point of view. Those so-called Tamasic humans, may do great damage to our environment, as their point of view is always 'bad/ugly' and their emotions are ruled by fear and aggression. Nevertheless, we must be brave and maintain our high level of confidence in the vision of Goodness and Beauty. No matter what happens, only our fortitude can be of help, not our despair.

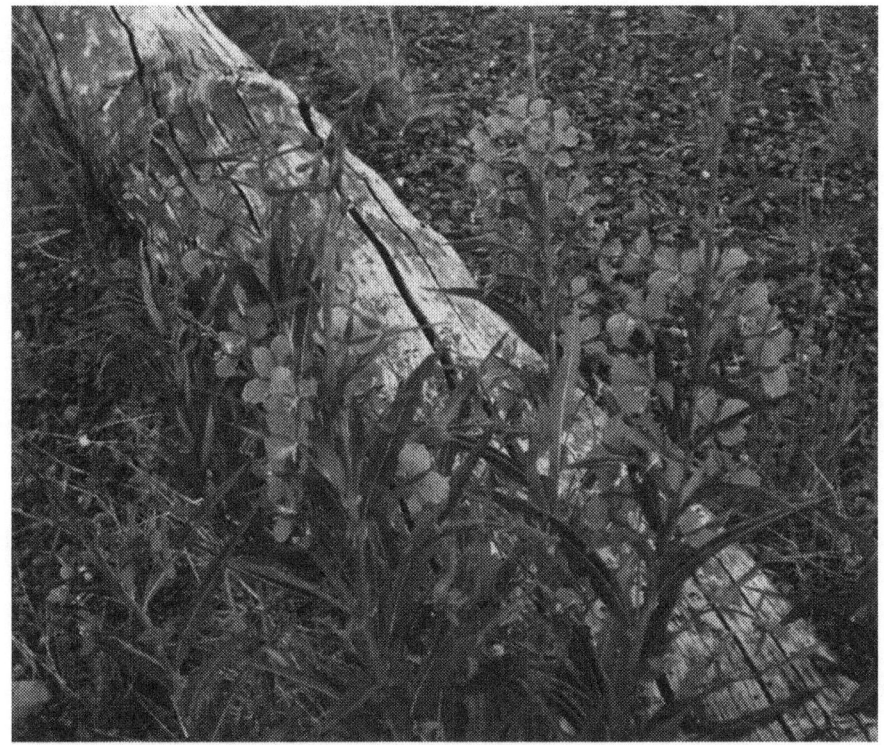

Flowers of the North

Re-incarnation and MAF

The subtle aspects of the events and their meaning in the Life of MAF.

MAF is an Italian female and is the reincarnation of a young Italian man called "Umberto." He was a Mason, a student of esoteric philosophy and mysticism, and a graduated student of medicine. Umberto was the fiancée of a young lady called Fanny and the close friend of her father who was also a Mason and a well-established medical professional.

When the First World War began in 1915, the military rules forced Umberto to go to war. Before leaving for the battlefield, he went to visit his dear fiancée Fanny and gave her the most precious little books that he was studying at that time: the books on Yoga by Yogi Ramacharaca printed in 1904. Later-on he was seriously wounded in the battlefield and died shortly after in a military camp. During his agony, Umberto maintained a strong desire to be reborn as a girl and as the daughter of Fanny. His intention was to continue to be in touch with Fanny and, being a girl, he would not be forced to participate in any future war. He wanted to be able to dedicate his new lifetime to the study of esoteric philosophies and to the practice of medicine, to help humanity.

The karma of the short life span and of the suffering of Umberto was determined by the fact that he was the reincarnation of a teenage girl who lived at the times of the Roman Empire.

One day, when MAF was a young girl, she had a clear vision of herself as a Roman teenager, sitting in a typical Roman patio, with a comforting lady at her side who was certainly Adeline. She was crying and coughing constantly because of her advanced pulmonary tuberculosis. During her agony, the Roman girl had a strong desire to die, as her short life had been very painful, oppressed, battered, and abused as a female. At death, her strong wish was to escape life and eventually to be a man, so that she could take revenge on those who had abused her.

As her karma was very heavy with bitterness, hatred and death desire, when she manifested again as Umberto, he could not live long. He had to suffer a painful death because of the deep resentments nurtured during the previous incarnation and still present at the moment of the previous transition. Nevertheless, Umberto had greatly improved the karma of that incarnating-Soul, by dedicating his attention to the study of medicine with the intention of helping others and therefore overcoming the ancient anger. He also practiced meditation and developed spiritual interests, evolving further in the purification of the manifesting-Soul.

The desire of Umberto at the moment of his death on the battlefield became reality when MAF was born as the daughter of Fanny, ten year later in 1925. However, there were strong contrasting powers and desires, as the father and the mother of MAF wanted a male, while the incarnating-Soul had been destined to be a female. The will of Destiny had to prevail, so, the presence of Adeline was required, and a furious icy storm was the needed event to complete the victory over opposing powers. It is possible that Adeline represented a nurturing entity dedicated to the evolution of that particular manifesting-Soul that lived the human life of the Roman girl, of Umberto and then of MAF. We cannot have the certainty of this aspect.

Once MAF was grown up and able to read, she was inspired to search in the house among the books of her mother Fanny and to find the booklets of Yogi Ramacharaka that were given for keeping to her by Umberto. This is what happened. Immediately, MAF felt a very strong attraction to these studies, even if she was only 9 years old. The practices of Yoga and of the breathing exercises were key elements to support her life, together with the caring presence of Adeline.

In the evolution of the Soul that incarnated in the form of MAF there was a lack of understanding of the importance, and of the meaning, of the five functions of the Cosmic Creating Consciousness. During the first decades of her human life, MAF could not grasp the significance of the interaction and alternation of Creation, Maintenance, Dissolution (or Destruction), Concealment, and Grace that are the constant flow of Divine Manifestation. This incapacity to understand made her deeply suffer. Suffering is needed to search for the Truth and to evolve.

The karmic destiny of MAF was to suffer greatly for not understanding the Cosmic Act of Dissolution and Renewal represented by the wars. MAF perceived only the physical aspect of the cruelty and destruction and could not conceive these as being an expression of Divine Will. War and devastation were needed to eradicate the large amount of hatred, resentment and desire of revenge that had accumulate on the continent of Europe after twenty years of dictatorships.

The emotional unbalance, the incapacity to cope, together with the physical irradiation of the neck at age eight, brought about the karmic cancer of thyroid at age forty. *MAF needed a strong shock to wake up!*

The cancer was karmic in the sense that it was a family karma shared by many members of the family. From the scientific point of view we would say that there was a genetic predisposition as several ancestors had died of cancer from both, the mother and father side. The particular point is that MAF did not die of it, as she should have. Other factors intervened.

As soon as MAF was born from her physical mother, the two powerful karmic Desires clashed. One was the desire for manifestation and Life, transmitted to the new incarnating-Soul as the last wish of the dying Umberto; the other karmic desire was for death, for not being a male, as the powerful want of both parents. The presence of a more evolved Soul, able to manifest Unconditional Love, was essential to determine the solution of the struggle. Adeline was that evolved-Soul and she was able to protect the growing child and teach her the essential "Unconditional Love" that the parent were not in condition to provide. The presence of Anne, her teachings, and the symbolic encounter with the statue of Jesus the Sheppard, were also important elements that prepared the girl for the intuition of searching and finding the three booklets on Yoga that Umberto gave to Fanny. The booklets were: Fourteen Lessons on Yoga, The Science of Breath, and Mystical Christianity by Yogi Ramacharaka. These typed booklets permitted the continuation of the learning exactly where the war and the final transition of Umberto interrupted them.

When at the age of forty invasive cancer became manifest and death was close, MAF underwent the fundamental crisis called "The dark night of the Soul." The

Christian Mystic, Juan of the Cross, in Spain, first used this definition. This necessary step helps the evolving-Soul to abandon any attachment to the body and to worldly desires. The profound sense of separation and loneliness is unbearable. The Soul becomes Self-conscious and cry: "I am alone and the whole universe is against me!"

Humans cannot endure this condition. The serious search for the Divine Self becomes an immediate necessity. Adeline was not there to help anymore. She had gone into transition two years before, but her teachings persisted; her Unconditional Love emerged from the depth of the subconscious and MAF received Grace and Will to overcome from the power of Adeline's Love.

Still, a concrete understanding of the "*injustice*" of war was needed and the answer to the question "*Who am I?*" was also urgent.

MAF had to struggle and wait several years to finally find the satisfactory answers. The Higher Self provided them, through the blessings of the great Sage Swami Muktananda Paramahamsa, in Ganeshpury, India.

Then, five years more of solitary confinement, meditation, yoga, breathing routines, silence and prayers were needed to incorporate all the new teachings and the profound change of universal perceptions. The Soul finally emerged full of Joy, entered permanent Bliss, and started to Live in Eternity at every terrestrial moment.

This was the complete change of MAF from an evolving-Soul to a Conscious-Soul, functioning as the Witness and not as a personal entity.

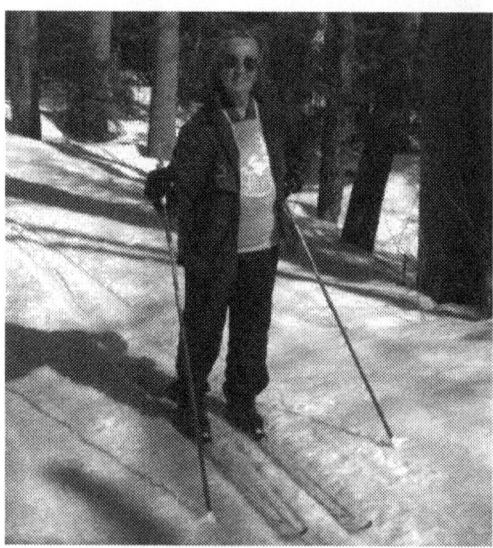

enjoying winter sports

Peace of soul and body in the new house in the woods

My younger son gave me a big surprise! He phoned me, and told me to find for him a new built house with at least "3 tall trees" around the house. It was not difficult. I went to a little town in Northern Ontario and found a beautiful property with twenty acres of woods, lots of tall trees, a pond, and a house recently built.

He bought it and I came to live in it.

Here I am, enjoying the tall maples, the spruces, the deer, the raccoons, and lots of birds. I keep busy with my daily spiritual practices of meditation and chanting and doing some pottery. Almost every day, in every season I am taking long walks in the pristine forest, breathing deeply the scent of old tress, chanting loud to answer the birds' call and enjoying the freedom of a true natural environment.

I give talks on Vibrational medicine and other Holistic heath topics.

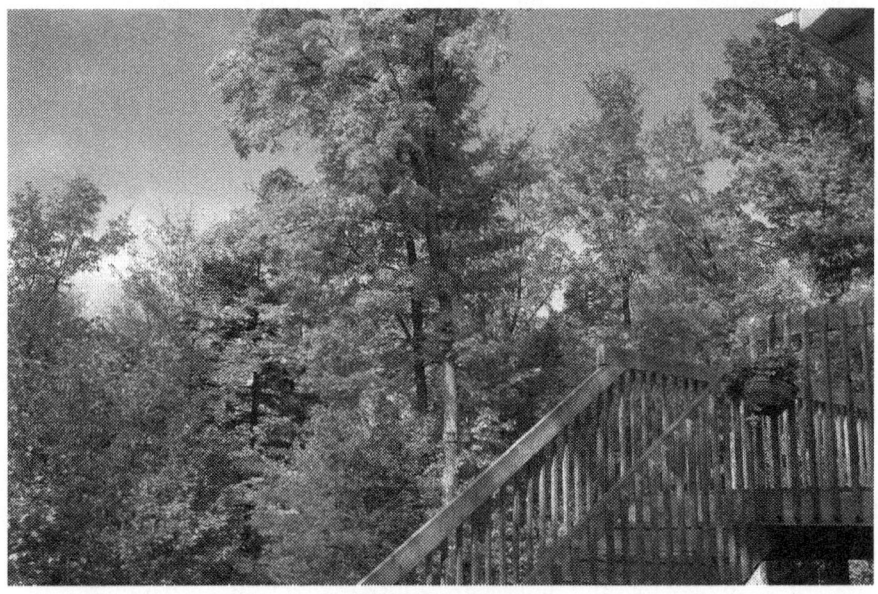

new house in the fall

Daily routine to stay active, happy, and strong.

I like to be alone and in silence. I sit in my easy chair and contemplate the sky and the trees from my living room; this in an essential activity that makes me happy and fulfilled. I am in touch with the wind and the movements of the branches, with the birds passing-by and with the clouds running in the sky. I usually completely ignore the rest of the world; I have already done all I could for society. Now, is my time to rest and deeply enjoy life in itself, without added movements or distractions. Solitude and silence are a gift of God!

I exercise daily in one way or another. About twice a week, in every season, I walk on a trail in the woods along a small river for one or two hours, covering about four kilometres. During these walks, I breathe very deeply, absorbing the energy of the forest and of the river; I return home completely refreshed!

On other days I do Tai chi, the set of 108 movements twice in a row; or I use a gym-machine that provides training for both legs and arms, doing two sets of ten minutes each, going as fast as possible.

Twice a week I use the 'chi-machine' and the 'far-infrared-dome' for about twenty to forty minutes, then I drink a lot of water! Almost every day I do acupressure or acupuncture in order to maintain the biological balance of the system; the channels of flowing energy must be free of obstructions!

My diet is based on brown rice, vegetables, and fruits. It is very easy to cook a large quantity of vegetable soup and store it in the freezer; the daily soup is then prepared by adding to it the delicious brown rice, fresh cooked in the special rice-cooking device. Apples, bananas, and a glass of milk complete the simple diet. No danger of gaining or loosing weight! I also take vitamins supplements regularly.

Daily rituals and worship are an important aspect of my life; chanting, meditation and the reading of sutras or sacred scriptures. I follow my Guru's advice: "Keep the company of saints!" and I am always in perfect company!

As entertainments I do some work of pottery, I give talks about health and vibrational medicine, and now I am writing this book. This is a long entertainment!

I also like to take pictures and I have a nice digital camera that goes with me everywhere; mostly when my sons invite me to go on vacation to the beach in the Caribbean or to the beach in California.

I am always grateful to the Divine Cosmic Consciousness for all the gifts that I receive! Peace and blessings to All!

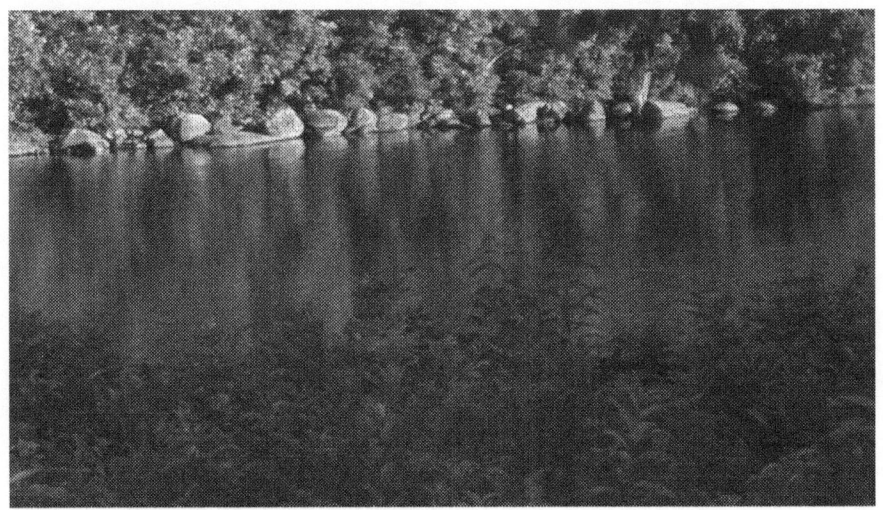

meditation lake

Conclusions

"Things are as they are because in no other way can they BE"

When everything goes well, we read this sentence and think, "Yes, it is ok!"

When things do not go well, then, it is a statement that is hard to swallow. In this case, if we are able to think big and perceive the wholeness of the universal connectivity, we will realize that whatever is not as it should be, must be changed or destroyed in order to function with all the rest.

The communication across the universe is instantaneous, much faster than the speed of light; the entangled subatomic particles are infinite in number and are able to transmit information instantly.

The smallest object has a certain influence on the whole. Our thoughts are real 'objects'; like wind and temperature, we cannot 'grasp' them with our hands; nevertheless, they are concrete objects with power of their own. If this would not be true, then all the discourse about our intentions would be meaningless.

In worldly legal matters, at the Court, the accused is judged according to the intention that guided the criminal act; the killing may be accidental or premeditate. The related sentence will be very different in each case. This shows that, in social and legal matters, the individual intention is what counts.

In the same way, the intention of groups of human beings will modify—something—at universal scale. What we call 'progress' comes about because most people want to live a more comfortable life. This desire produces a change, not only in the lives of the population, but on the conditions of the entire universe.

The above sentence: "All Things are as they are because in no other way can they BE", is not a judgment of something good or bad; it only states that, no matter what happens, the main attribute of the universe is to 'exist', 'BE'. Therefore, it will globally bring about the conditions that best fit this 'being'.

The essential unit of the manifested universe is 'vibration'. The ancient Seers of India more than ten thousand years ago understood that all is vibration. They named Spanda, the first, very subtle vibration that emanated from the Absolute. All the manifested universes derive from Spanda. The universal vibrations are Light, Goodness, and Beauty. Humanity evolves and expands in harmony with the cosmic vibrations, finds synchronization and fulfillment in them. They are reality and the true essence of all.

Our humanity, as we know it on the Planet Earth is not the only manifested humanity, in the sense of evolved, intelligent and self-conscious beings. Many other groups are scattered on million of celestial bodies. Scientific research has confirmed that our universe is particularly adapted to the presence and development of Life. Therefore, there are certainly self-conscious beings somewhere in our universe. We all are one unit.

If humanity understands its close participation in the universal whole and behaves in harmony with it, all will go well and the human race may exist and prosper for extended periods. On the contrary, if populations become a threat to the global well-being, they will be instantly erased.

This is the profound warning suggested by the sentence:
All Things are as they are because in no other way can they BE.

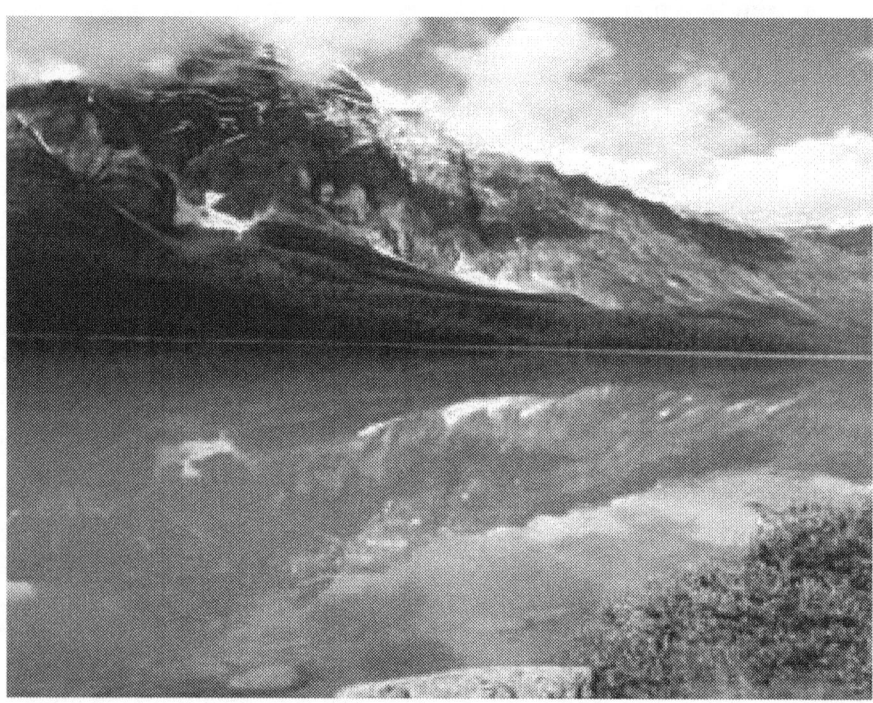

Lake in the Canadian Rockies

My closing message

Now, read my little poem and try to understand what I *really* mean!
My intention is to pay a tribute to Life, Love, and Freedom.

> After we reject everything else, only Love is left.
> Love exists even when we try to reject it.
> In the same way, we cannot pull ourselves away
> From the attraction of the Sun.
> The Sun is always there, even if we don't see it,
> Because of some clouds.
> The Sun of our Life is within us all the time,
> However, sometimes we may not perceive it's shining.
>
> During times of war, dark clouds cover our landscape.
> We wander in a wasteland of despair.
> The giants of fear, hatred, frustration and revenge,
> Are powerful and menacing.
> During times of peace, the sun is shining over our future.
> We hear the distant echoes of joy, hope, and reassurance.
> We feel aligned with all creation,
> We belong and we shine.
>
> But, as life goes on, alternating the times,
> The ups and the downs,
> We come to understand that all is a play,
> All comes and goes, like waves at seashore.
>
> All is a rhythmic motion that we can watch
> With a distant interest and a caring look.
> When we achieve real detachment, we merge
> In the glory of True Love Unconditional.
>
> Separation from the Source of Life,
> Is our weakness and our doubt.
>
> Desire to Know, is the motivation for our Quest.
> Experience of Union, is finally our Certainty.

Love for our-selves,
Understanding for all.

Wisdom and Compassion are the pillars
Of Human Divine Consciousness.

∧∧∧∧∧∧∧∧∧∧∧∧∧∧∧∧∧

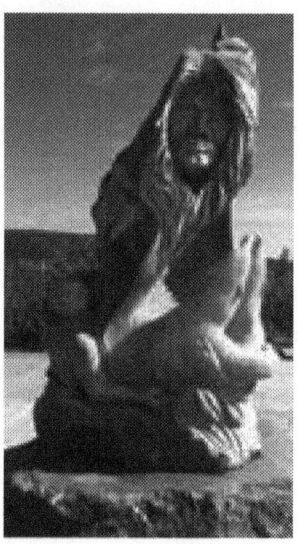

Art of the Inuit's, Symbolic sculpture …

Bibliography

Avaduta Gita	India, Madras: Sri Ramakrishna Math, 1981
Avalon Arthur	*The Serpent Power,* New York: Dover Publications, Inc., 1958.
BAGAVAD GITA	South Africa, Durban: Sivananda Press, The Divine Light Society, 1968.
BUDDHA	*Dhammapada,* Mexico: Editorial Diana,1970.
Campbell Joseph	*Oriental Mythology,* New York: Penguin Books, 1962.
Cleary Thomas	*The Taoist Classics,* Boston: Shambala, 2003.
	The Taoist I Ching, Boston: Shambala, 1986.
	The Taoist I Ching Mandalas, Boston: Shambhala, 1989.
Colins Mabel	*Ligth on the Path,* New York: Kessinger Publishing, 1911.
Dyczkowski Mark	*The Doctrine of Vibration,* Albany: State University of NY, Press, 1987.
Farhi Donna	*The Breathing book,* New York: Henry Holt and Co.,LLC, 1996.
Gerber Richard, M.D.	*Vibrational Medicine,* Vermont: Bear & Co., third edition, 2001.
Maoshing Ni, Ph.D.	*The yellow Emperor's Classic of medicine,* Boston: Shambhala, 1995.
Muktananda Swami	*Chitshakti Vilas,* Ganeshpury, India: Gurudev Siddha Peeth, 1978.
	Reflections of the Self, Gurudev Siddha Peeth, 1980
	Light on the Path, Gurudev Siddha Peeth, 1981.
	The perfect relationship, Gurudev Siddha Peeth, 1980.
	Paramartha Katha Prasang, Gurudev Siddha Peeth, 1981.
	Does Death really exist? Gurudev Siddha Peeth, 1981.
	Satsang with Baba vol.one Gurudev Siddha Peeth, 1974.
	Satsang with Baba vol.two Gurudev Siddha Peeth, 1976.
	Satsang with Baba vol. five Gurudev Siddha Peeth, 1978.
	Secret of The Siddhas, Gurudev Siddha Peeth, 1980.
	I Am That, SYDA Foundation, NY, 1992.
PATANJALI	*Yoga philosophy,* Albany: State University of NY Press, 1983.

Ramacharaka Yogi   *Yogi Philosophy*, New York:The Yoga Publication Society, 1931.
Mystic Christianity, New York: Kessinger Publishing, LLC, 1907.

Reed Gach M. Ph.D. *Acupressure's Potent Points*, New York: Bantam Book, 1990.
Acupresure for Emotional Healing, New York: Bantam Book, 2004.

Rosenblum B., et Al. *Quantum enigma*, Oxford: Oxford University Press, 2006.

Schroedinger Erwin *What is Life?* Cambridge: Cambridge University Press, fifth printing, 2006.

Shantanada Swami   *The splendor of Recognition*, New York: SYDA Foundations, 2003.

Siddha Yoga   *Meditation Revolution*, New York: Agama Press, 1997.

Singh Jaideva   *Pratyabhijnahrdayam*, Delhi, India: Motilal Banarsidass, 1980.
Siva Sutras, Delhi, India: Motilal Banarsidass, 1979.
Spanda Karika, Delhi, India: Motilal Banarsidass, 1980.
Vijnanabhairava, Delhi, India: Motilal Banarsidass, 1979.

VenkatesanandaSwami *Vasistha's Yoga*, New York: State University of NY Press, 1993.

Wilber Ken   *The holographic Paradigm*, Boston: Shambhala Pub. 1982.
Quantum Questions, Boston: Shambhala Pub. 2001.

Wilhelm Hellmut   *Understanding the I Ching*, Princeton University Press,1995.

Wilhelm Richard   *The I Ching*, Princeton: Princeton University Press,1975, 12th printing.

Wing R. L.   *The Illustrated I Ching*, New York: Bantam Pub., 1982
The Tao of Power, New York: Bantam Pub., 1986.

Yogananda Swami   *Autobiography of a Yogi*, Bombay: Jaico Publishing, 1980.

Zukav Gary   *The Dancing Wu Li Masters*, New York: Bantam Books, 1979.

978-0-595-42531-0
0-595-42531-3